Compartments

Compartments

*How the Brightest, Best Trained, and
Most Caring People Can Make Judgments
That are Completely and Utterly Wrong*

Steven R. Feldman, MD, PhD

*Professor of Dermatology, Pathology,
and Public Health Sciences*

Wake Forest University School of Medicine

Library of Congress Control Number:		2009903274
ISBN:	Hardcover	978-1-4415-2633-5
	Softcover	978-1-4415-2632-8

To order additional copies of this book, contact:
Xlibris Corporation
1-888-795-4274
www.Xlibris.com
Orders@Xlibris.com
60224

Contents

Preface

Why is there so much conflict in our world? Is there an evil power that creates conflict? Depending on how you look at it, the answer may be yes. This book presents stories of the common misjudgments and conflicts that occur every day between groups of people in our health care system and other organizations. Most people can easily relate to these problems and to the similar issues in their own lives. This book illustrates core principles about conflict that should be considered whenever we think about people in other groups:

(1) There are things we don't see.
(2) There are things we see that we should not trust.
(3) Context affects our perceptions.

These three principles underlie much of the conflict we find in the world around us.

Introduction

There are many great people in our country, caring people, with a vision for the future. These people are committed to the principles on which this country was founded, principles of freedom and of equality. People like John McCain, Barack Obama, and Mike Huckabee come to mind as well as Cal Thomas, Jane Fonda, Charlton Heston, Phyllis Schlafly, Gloria Steinem, Jesse Helms, and Al Franken. These people—and probably you too—are people of principle, people who believe in working to make the world a better place.

Though all these people have ideals based on a strong moral foundation, they don't all quite see the world in the same way . . . not by a long shot. The different views they hold aren't because some of them are bright and some of them are stupid. These are all bright people. And the differences aren't because some of them are good, caring people and some of them are evil, bad people. These are all idealists, people who have a commitment to basic principles that we might all agree on. Why do they and so many other people see the world in such different ways?

We live in worlds that are compartmentalized. Often, we find conflict between these compartments. There are rivalries between schools, even rivalries between fraternities within schools.

Different divisions of a company may be at odds. While we expect conflict between different armies, there is often conflict between the different branches of a single country's armed forces. In the medical world, there is conflict between doctors and other health care providers, between health care providers and insurers, and even between different specialties of physicians. There are rivalries, and even violence, between people of different religions and between countries.

What causes these conflicts? Is one side good, and the other side evil? The premise of this book is that the compartmentalization of our world results in misunderstanding and conflict. The borders of the compartments in which we live our lives cause tremendous misunderstanding. Sometimes we are completely prevented from knowing what is happening in another compartment. Even when we do see what is happening in another compartment, sometimes our observations aren't representative of what is normal in that other compartment. Moreover, there are indirect effects of compartments, such that even if we "see" accurate representations of another compartment, our perceptions of what we see may be deeply affected by the context in which we view the observation. The borders of the compartments in which we live our lives are like blinders that obscure reality in fundamentally powerful and insidious ways.

Understanding compartments and how they affect our perceptions has important implications for how we view the world around us. These implications are so profound they may challenge many of the concepts we have been taught, even those that previously have been confirmed by our own personal observations of the world around us. Some of the implications may be so at odds with how we currently view things as to seem goofy or perhaps even dangerous. These are the ones where it is probably most important to reconsider our closely held views.

By understanding the sources of misunderstanding, we can better position ourselves to end conflict. The sources of misunderstanding that occur between individuals on a daily basis are not altogether different from the sources of international conflict between peoples and nations. By recognizing the effects of the compartments in which we live our lives, we can have a better understanding of our world and end many of the conflicts, which we face.

PART 1

Things We Do Not See

You Can't Trust What You Don't See

Perhaps the best thing about being a doctor is seeing a suffering patient get well under your care. One of the most frustrating things about being a doctor is caring for a patient and not seeing him or her get any better. Often, patients do great. Sometimes, they don't. Sometimes, the treatment just doesn't work nearly as well as expected. And sometimes even when the treatment does well at first, after a while it doesn't. In fact, one of the basic principles of my specialty, dermatology, is that after a while, the most commonly used medications—topical cortisone medicines—simply stop working.

The discovery of cortisone in 1948 revolutionized medicine and secured the 1950 Nobel Prize in Medicine for the discoverers, Philip Hench, Edward Kendall, and Tadeusz Reichstein. Kendall, a chemist, described the impact of the new medication: "On September 21, 1948, cortisone was administered to a patient who had rheumatoid arthritis. During the preceding five years she had continued to become worse and at the time that cortisone was given she was confined to her bed and endured much pain. Within a week she walked out of the hospital in a gay mood and went on a shopping trip for three hours without after effects" (Kendall 1953). As effective as cortisone was, even more powerful derivatives were created soon after. In the 1950s, cortisone formulations were developed that could be rubbed on the skin. These topical medications—medications applied to the skin—dramatically changed how skin diseases were treated.

While topical cortisone medicines provided a tremendous advance in the treatment of skin disease, their tendency to lose effectiveness over time limited their usefulness. This was a particularly difficult problem for people with chronic, incurable conditions like the one I specialize in treating: psoriasis. Psoriasis is a condition that causes red, scaly spots on the body. It is usually treated with topical cortisone medicines. The eventual loss of efficacy of topical cortisone treatments is so common and well characterized that it has a name: *tachyphylaxis*. Teachers of dermatology have, for generations, taught their students that tachyphylaxis can be defined as "the more you use the medicine, the less it works."

Various treatment approaches were used to minimize the tachyphylaxis problem. Sometimes doctors would prescribe topical cortisone medicines to be used intermittently so the patient's disease wouldn't get used to the medicine. Sometimes treatments would be rotated from one approach to another in order to prevent patients from getting used to a particular treatment.

The concept of tachyphylaxis is simple enough. As people continue to use strong cortisone medicines, tolerance develops, and the medicine eventually loses effectiveness. Cortisone drugs work by binding to cortisone receptors in the skin. The loss of effectiveness makes perfect sense if continued exposure to cortisone causes the receptors for cortisone to disappear or to become less sensitive to the drug over time. This receptor desensitization theory provided a good explanation of why people who used the medication for long periods eventually developed tolerance to the drug.

But one thing didn't quite fit the theory. If a patient became resistant to one cortisone drug, the doctor could prescribe a cortisone of a different brand—yet still of the same potency level—and the new drug would work just fine. The doctor didn't necessarily need to prescribe a higher-strength cortisone. If patients had become resistant to topical cortisone because their cortisone receptors were reduced in number or in function, changing the brand of the cortisone should not have overcome the tolerance that had developed.

A small, simple research study turned theories about the loss of efficacy of topical treatments upside down. In the study, patients with psoriasis were given a gel to apply (6 percent salicylic acid gel, a safe medication commonly used to remove the thick scales that cover psoriasis spots) (Carroll 2004). The patients were told to use the medication twice a day. They were told that their use of the medication would be monitored, and they were asked to complete a daily diary of their use of the medicine. They also were asked to bring the medication back at return visits so the medication could be weighed. They were *not* told, however, that there were computer chips in the medication bottle caps recording their use of the medicine. Those computer chips didn't just record the number of times the medication bottles were opened; the monitors recorded the day and time each time the bottle was opened or closed to see when patients actually used the medication.

The study found that the patients overreported their use of the medication (and that's being generous). Some patients who hardly used the medicine at all recorded using it almost exactly as had been directed. One of the most important and interesting findings was that the use of the medication dropped steadily over time. Although the patients claimed they had been using the medication regularly as instructed, use of the medication dropped by about 20 percent every five weeks. The study lasted a total of eight weeks. We can't know for sure what would have happened to the use of the medication after the eight-week study, but if that decrease in the rate of use continued, patients could be expected to stop using the medication entirely in twenty-five weeks or in about six months.

Dermatologists prescribe patients medications but don't get to see what patients do with the medicines. Doctors prescribe in one compartment—their offices; patients use the medications in another compartment—at home. It had long been assumed that because patients' skin disease bothers them that they would use their medications. It turns out many patients don't use their topical medications as directed, and over the long run, their use of medication steadily drops. But dermatologists didn't know this. Dermatology textbooks didn't say anything about patients not using their medications.

Theories about how medications lose effectiveness over time changed completely. Dermatologists originally thought tachyphylaxis was "the more you use the medication, the less it works." But tachyphylaxis was really, "the less you use the medication, the less it works." Generations of brilliant professors of dermatology had been teaching their students the wrong thing, and generations of students of dermatology had accepted the traditional concepts. Dermatologists had no way of knowing that patients weren't using their medicines until the development of electronic monitors in medication bottle caps.

The electronic evidence of patients' use (or nonuse) of their medication didn't just change theories about tachyphylaxis. Theories about all sorts of other dermatologic phenomena went kaput (Ali 2007). There was the phenomenon of children with eczema—an itchy, dry skin condition—that wouldn't get better despite all attempts at outpatient management (Krejci-Manwaring 2007). These patients wouldn't improve despite the use of potent topical or even oral medications. If the frustration with treatment and the severity of disease mounted high enough, these patients would be admitted to the hospital for treatment of the intractable skin disease. They would be treated with rather modest topical treatments, and they would clear up dramatically in just two or three days! For a long time dermatologists taught that these children probably did better in the hospital because they were away from the stress of the home environment, as if trying to sleep in a hospital bed is less stressful for a child than sleeping in his or her own bed at home. Now we know that hospitalized children with eczema improve so quickly because in the hospital someone ensures that the medication is applied as prescribed.

There had been so much dogma about skin diseases and their treatment that was patently ridiculous, and it was built up like a house of cards. All these ideas depended on the assumption that patients use their medications as directed. But you can't depend on assumptions that you can't test. A whole host of theories can be wrong, collapsing under the weight of a single inaccurate assumption. Learned teachers—even though they were brilliant, caring, and honest—could be completely mistaken.

We ought to be circumspect when we try to draw conclusions about things of which we don't have firsthand knowledge. The immortal words of Donald Rumsfeld come to mind (Seely 2003):

> As we know, there are known knowns. There are things we
> know we know. We also know there are known unknowns.
> That is to say, we know there are some things we do not
> know. But there are also unknown unknowns, the ones
> we don't know we don't know.

We recognize that known unknowns are a problem. Rumsfeld cautions us that there may also be unknown unknowns that may cause us to stumble. But perhaps our biggest problem may be that the things we know we know just aren't true.

Why Are They Doing That?

Doctors don't always know why patients behave the way they do. One of my most memorable patients in this regard had a condition that wasn't particularly out of the ordinary. She was a single woman, about thirty years old, and she looked like she was in her late 40s. She was a tanner, a frequent tanner.

Perhaps you know people like her, people who use tanning beds so often that their skin has become mottled, wrinkled, or even leathery. People tan to look good, but frequent tanners' skin looks terrible (think of Magda in the Farrelly brothers' *There's Something About Mary*).

My memorable patient was a bright, energetic young woman who worked as a health care professional. When she came in, she was worried about a lesion on her chest that might have been a skin cancer. Just doing a biopsy on the spot was going to leave an unsightly scar. But she was still tanning. We know that people tan so they can look better, so why don't these tanners stop when the tanning makes them look so bad? Why do they do it when they know tanning can cause skin cancer?

Tanning has become an enormous mom-and-pop industry in the United States and various other parts of the world. Tanning bed establishments have popped up everywhere. In crossroad towns so small that there's just a stop sign with a gas station on the corner, there's usually a tanning bed in the back of the gas station. Some of the most voracious tanners get their own tanning bed to use at home.

The health careers teacher at one of our local high schools was concerned about how much tanning the girls in her class were doing. The prom was approaching, and many of her students had already been to a tanning bed numerous times. The health career teacher, who had previously worked as a nurse in my dermatology office, had me come speak to her class.

There were fifteen students in the class—all girls. I expected that two or three of these girls had been to a tanning salon but was shocked to find that every student in that health careers course with the exception of one (an olive-skinned Latino girl who wanted to look lighter) was actively tanning. Many of the girls had red and burned faces the day I visited caused by their last tanning visit. These were students in a health careers class. They had been doing internships at nursing homes and had seen firsthand the wrinkles and the skin cancers caused by ultraviolet radiation. Still, they were tanning. A few were tanning every day.

I understand that teenagers don't tend to worry much about the future. To them, the risk of skin cancer in later life is of almost no importance. What matters to them is how they look, how they are perceived by their friends now, and how they think their friends perceive them. Despite the beautiful pictures of Nicole Kidman and Julianne Moore on the cover of magazines, our society still tells kids that dark is in. The social pressure gets people to start tanning. But that doesn't explain why frequent tanners continue their tanning when the wrinkles, the mottled color, and the leathery feel of their skin begin to show.

Researchers studied the phenomenon, looking at "appearance motivation" and how it drove people to tanning beds. Researchers studied the social pressures to look good. They tried developing ways to get people to stop the excessive tanning. Telling patients about skin cancer risks didn't help. One study found that tanners knew more about skin cancer than nontanners (Mawn 1993). Tanning sprays came out that could make a person look dark without injuring the skin, but people still exposed themselves to ultraviolet light. In fact, tanning establishments began adding newer "turbo" beds that put out even more ultraviolet radiation. Dermatologists were living in a different compartment than frequent tanners and had no idea of the real reason the frequent tanners—those tanners who had made their skin look old and ugly by societal standards—were tanning so much.

The explanation came from an unexpected source. Dr. Mina Yaar and her colleagues at Boston University were studying suntans (Wintzen 1996). When ultraviolet light hits skin, a skin cell called the melanocyte makes melanin, the pigment that makes our skin dark. More melanin in the skin is what gives us a suntan. Yaar was trying to understand how ultraviolet light causes skin cells to produce more melanin.

Dr. Yaar exposed skin cells in the laboratory to ultraviolet light. The cells made a hormone called melanocyte-stimulating hormone, MSH. The production of MSH helps explain how ultraviolet light causes a suntan. But Yaar found something else too. The production of MSH was paired with the production of endorphin, the natural "feel good" molecule of the body. Endorphins bind and activate the same receptors that bind drugs like morphine and heroin.

Ultraviolet light didn't just make the hormone for a suntan; it also made the hormone that makes people feel good. Yaar's work offered an explanation for why people go to the beach (and not to caverns) on their vacations. Her work explained why beaches are full of people in the middle of the day when the damaging rays are at their worst. Her work offered the first explanation of why

---

frequent tanners were continuing to damage their skin despite knowing it was making them look old and wrinkled.

My colleagues and I did an experiment to test whether frequent tanners were driven to tan by the way ultraviolet light made them feel, not by the way tanning made them look (Feldman 2004). We enrolled frequent tanners, people who were tanning three times a week or more, in our study. In the experiment, the frequent tanners tanned in two tanning beds. These were state-of-the-art commercial tanning beds, the ones most widely used in the United States. One bed was a normal tanning bed that gave UV light. The other was designed to look identical in every way except that there was no UV.[1]

The frequent tanners had tanning sessions in both tanning beds on Monday and again on Wednesday. The tanners couldn't tell which bed was giving them a tan because they were exposed to both beds, one immediately after the other on both days. On Friday the tanners were given the opportunity to tan again, and they could choose which of the two beds in which to do it. Almost invariably (95 percent of the time) they chose the bed that gave them the ultraviolet light.

---

[1] In these beds, tanners lie on a clear plastic sheet made of acrylic, protecting them from the bulbs underneath. There are different types of acrylics. One of the tanning beds in the experiment used the acrylic that is normally used in tanning beds, an acrylic that lets ultraviolet light pass through. The second bed used an ultraviolet-blocking acrylic, the kind people would normally use for framing a picture to hang near a window; the ultraviolet-blocking acrylic helps keep ultraviolet light from bleaching the picture. Both acrylics let visible light pass through, so they look the same, but only one of the acrylics lets the ultraviolet light pass through. The bed with the ultraviolet-blocking acrylic was a control bed. It looked identical to the ultraviolet bed in every way, but it didn't give the tanners any ultraviolet light.

The experiment had been "blinded." We didn't tell the tanners which bed had ultraviolet and which bed didn't. But the tanners could tell. The two beds felt different to them. The bed that gave the ultraviolet light gave the tanners a greater sense of relaxation, the feeling of relaxation one gets from lying out at the beach on a summer's day. The sense of relaxation doesn't come just from the heat. There is no industry of quiet, dark, warm closets that people pay to use. Nor do most people lie out at the beach on pleasantly warm summer nights. The beach is crowded with people during the stinking-hottest part of the day when ultraviolet light is at its maximum. The relaxation people feel, especially the relaxation the frequent tanners experience, comes from the effect of the ultraviolet light on their skin.

Additional studies have confirmed that the frequent tanners are driven to tan by more than just appearance. One group of researchers studied beachgoers and found that, like alcoholics, there is an addictive pattern to tanning (Warthan 2005). Another group of researchers studied college students and found that the most frequent tanners exhibited a pathological tendency to tan (Hillhouse 2007).

We further tested the theory that natural endorphins drive frequent tanning in a small pilot study using the endorphin blocker naltrexone. If someone were to come to an emergency room overdosed on heroin or morphine, a doctor might give the patient an endorphin blocker like naltrexone to reverse the effects of the overdose. If frequent tanning was driven by release of endorphin, then giving an endorphin blocker would block frequent tanners' ability to distinguish the tanning bed that gave ultraviolet light from the one that didn't.

In a preliminary study, we gave three frequent tanners naltrexone prior to the tanning bed exposures (Kaur 2005). The naltrexone blocked the preference for ultraviolet light in the first subject, but in the next two, something unexpected happened. These two subjects felt sick. They felt nauseous and jittery. Naltrexone isn't supposed to make normal people sick. But it does have that effect on people who are chronically addicted to narcotics. The subjects had their urine tested for narcotics use, and they were clean. It seemed that these frequent tanners were showing signs of withdrawal, of being addicted to the effects of the ultraviolet light. The findings were confirmed in a larger study of eight frequent tanners and eight people who had tried tanning but who didn't tan on a regular basis (Kaur 2006). People in each group were exposed in both tanning beds. During these tanning sessions, subjects received either the naltrexone medication or a placebo substitute. None of the subjects getting placebo felt sick. None of the infrequent tanners got sick. Half the frequent tanners developed symptoms (like nausea and jitteriness) suggestive of a withdrawal reaction.

Frequent tanners tan themselves because of how it makes them feel. Some do it to the point of addiction. Dermatologists, however, thought that frequent tanners had been tanning because of how it made them look. Dermatologists thought the problem was that frequent tanners were trying to look dark. That didn't really make sense. People who were tanning this much didn't just look dark; they looked terrible—wrinkled, mottled, leathery. There had to be another reason why these people were tanning, but dermatologists couldn't see it from their own perspective. Dermatologists were in one compartment and made erroneous assumptions about people in another compartment. Dermatologists didn't and couldn't see that the real reason the frequent tanners were tanning so much was because of how it made them feel, because of an "addiction" to the ultraviolet light.

Dermatologists probably could have talked among themselves forever and not figured out what the frequent tanners already knew—that tanning gives these frequent tanners a pleasant sense of relaxation and that this sense of relaxation is a major reason these frequent tanners are tanning so much. When people in one group (or compartment) are trying to understand people in a second group, it often helps if they would just talk (and listen) to one another. If dermatologists had asked frequent tanners why they were doing this to themselves, tanners would have told the dermatologists how relaxing tanning is. Many times, we have to look past the compartment we're in to find out how things really are in another compartment.

Other Things We Just Can't See

The world is organized in compartments. This doesn't just apply to dermatologists and their patients. It applies to all of us and the world around us. Young people are separated into different schools. In business, people are organized into different divisions like sales, marketing, and business development. People in different countries live in different compartments. People of different faiths exist in different distinct groups. Everywhere we look we can find people separated into different compartments. People in one compartment often miss important aspects about people in another. Misperceptions are the usual result.

In a small medical office, employees may be divided in separate compartments, including scheduling/reception, billing, nursing, and physicians. People in each group may develop warped ideas about the other. Physicians may only notice the scheduling staff when there is a problem; such physicians may get the wrong idea that the scheduling staff isn't working hard or isn't committed to providing patients good service. Even if the physician recognizes that scheduling staff are doing great work most of the time, the physician may not comment about the staff's work unless there is a problem, leaving the scheduling staff with the mistaken impression that their boss doesn't appreciate their efforts. The misperceptions can poison office morale.

In large, compartmentalized organizations, conflicts are even more common. Consider how people with different roles in the armed forces perceive each other. The infantry works hard to stay in shape and readiness, and they probably think soldiers in supply have it easy. Soldiers in supply struggle with extraordinary complex logistical issues and probably think the infantry folks don't have enough to do. Large corporations face similar issues. The marketing department probably thinks that salespeople don't work hard enough and that "they can't execute." People in sales think the marketing folks are not productive and that "the marketing plan stinks." Rarely do people see how hard people are working in other compartments.

When people are in different groups, there are barriers to communication. The barriers may be physical, like walls and distance. The barriers can also be cultural or social ones that keep people from talking to one another. The barriers between different groups of people limit communication and our ability to know what is happening in another group. Often we end up with wrong ideas about other people. We may have teachers and leaders who are very smart and caring, yet if they are part of our group, they may not know any more than we do about people in other groups.

Trying to understand people in a different compartment is fraught with hazard. Without firsthand experience, it is very difficult to know what other people are doing or thinking. We can sometimes see other people's behavior, but we don't know what caused the behavior. If we are communicating with them, they can tell us why they did what they did. Frequently what other people are thinking is very different from what we imagine was going through their heads.

Take the example of incompetent automobile drivers. It is not uncommon to be upset by another driver on the road, someone who cut you off or who was driving too fast. Perhaps you wondered if they were drunk, incompetent, or just mean-spirited. It's possible they were. It's easy to get angry at people driving like that. What total disregard for others they *seem* to have. Of course, we don't really know what they are thinking. It could be there was something else going on. Maybe the other driver did not realize how they were affecting other people. Maybe they were on their way to the hospital with an emergency. Maybe they were lost. We can't know. We aren't in their car, much less in their head.

If you ever accidently did something that seemed stupid or bad to someone else, the other person may have misinterpreted your intent. We shouldn't assume evil intent on the part of another based on a superficial view of their actions. Generally, we shouldn't draw conclusions from data we don't have. It's better to ask and to listen than to assume we know why someone else behaved the way they did. More often than not, such communication alleviates workplace conflict.

Sometimes words alone don't seem to communicate very well, leaving plenty of room for miscommunication. In our modern world, e-mail is famous for this. While e-mail is an incredible tool for communication, a Google search of "e-mail and miscommunication" gives 700,000 hits. The potential for miscommunication with e-mail is enormous. Human conversation expresses itself in words, body language, inflection, and tone of voice. Words alone miss many of the cues we take for granted in our daily communication. Messages sent by e-mail from one compartment to another often don't adequately communicate what the sender intended.

Researchers Nicholas Epley and Justin Kruger investigated how people's expectations can affect their interpretation of e-mail messages (Epley 2005). The interpretation of e-mail messages was much more likely to be affected by preset biases and expectations than were interpretations of voice communications. The researchers suggested that e-mail messages are inherently more ambiguous than voice communication and that people communicating electronically tend to "fill in the blanks" with their expectations and stereotypes. In one of their experiments, they tested people's ability to detect sarcasm (Kruger 2005). They had college students read or e-mail sarcastic or nonsarcastic statements to other students. They measured how well the receivers recognized the sarcastic statements as sarcasm. The receivers were much better at recognizing sarcasm in voice communication than they were from e-mail messages. Importantly, the researchers demonstrated that people's egocentrism affected how they interpreted the messages they received.

You may have noticed the effects of e-mail miscommunication in your workplace or personal interactions. Senders know what they want to say, but receivers of messages generally interpret the words from their own perspective and with their own preconceived biases. Unintended slights and hurt feelings may result. Sometimes, the miscommunication gets blown totally out of proportion. The potential for miscommunication is even greater when there are language or cultural barriers that have to be overcome.

Compartments set us up for miscommunication. Talking to people—particularly when it is done in person—bridges the divide between compartments and helps reduce the opportunities for errors in communication and for misconceptions based on preconceived biases. Taking things at face value and making assumptions about why people act the way they do leaves far too much opportunity for errors in judgment.

Getting past the limitations of our compartments is essential to solving our most critical conflicts. Today, we face potential violence of horrific proportions from terrorists. To stop terrorism, we need to understand the terrorist. Compartments make that difficult. The terrorists belong to a different group. It would be very easy to have misconceptions about terrorists' motivations.

Some people say the terrorists hate us for our freedoms. Former President Bush said, "They hate our freedoms—our freedom of religion, our freedom of speech, our freedom to vote and assemble and disagree with each other"(Bush 2001). Bush is not one of the terrorists; he isn't a member of their compartment. Does he really know why the terrorists are attacking us? Does it make sense that they hate us for our freedom? We might wonder if that makes about as much sense as dermatologists thinking that messy cortisone medicines stopped working because of tolerance or that frequent tanners with mottled, wrinkled skin were tanning primarily because they liked the way it made them look.

It is painful to listen, but one of the terrorists tried to tell us why he hates us. Zacarias Moussaoui was convicted in March 2006 of conspiring to kill Americans as part of the September 11, 2001, terrorist attacks. At his sentencing, family members of the 9/11 victims confronted Moussaoui. In response, he said, "You said I destroyed a life and you lost a husband. Maybe one day you can think about how many people in the CIA have destroyed a life. You say we are a hate organization. I say [sarcastically] the CIA is a peace and love organization" (CNN 2006). Speaking to another family member of a 9/11 victim who was in the navy, Moussaoui went on to say, "Of course he was working for the government of peace and love on a *warship*. This country has hypocrisy beyond belief. Your humanity is selective. Only you suffer. Only you feel. You have branded me a terrorist or criminal. Look at yourself first . . . I have nothing more to say. You don't want to hear the truth. You wasted an opportunity for this country to know why people like me, why people like Mohamed Atta have so much hatred."

We need to know the real reasons that terrorists hate us. Based on the few words Moussaoui was permitted to speak, it doesn't appear he hates us for our freedom. On the contrary, it seems he hates us for committing the kind of violence and killing that we ourselves find abhorrent. Bin Laden says he hates us because of our support of Israel in the killing of Palestinians, because of America's troops stationed in Muslim countries, because of our support for dictators in Gulf states, and because of sanctions we imposed that resulted in the deaths of Arab children (Christian Science Monitor 2001; CNN 2004). Former President Bush says the terrorists hate us for our freedoms. To understand what terrorists are thinking, we may have to get past our compartment and listen to them rather than simply listening to ourselves.

A Golden Rule

One of the ways compartments cause conflict is by preventing us from seeing what's happening outside our compartment. Looking into the other compartment—getting to know the people in another compartment and what happens there—is the obvious solution. Businesses might do this by encouraging people from different departments to spend time together, for example by sending marketing staff out with salespeople to meet customers or by having sales staff spend some time working in marketing. Doctors can learn about patients' compartments by taking time to learn more about their patients' lives or perhaps by going back to the once-venerated home visit. Different religious groups may achieve greater interfaith understanding by performing shared charitable activities.

But compartments don't always lend themselves to direct observation. It is not always easy to see how people in other compartments think. We never get to see what is going on in someone else's head. Outside of mind readers and science fiction movies, the best we can do is to ask the other person what they are thinking. If we're lucky, they'll tell us and tell us honestly. But when we're not in a position to ask—for example, when it is someone or some group of people with whom we're not in direct contact—we simply cannot get behind the curtain to find out what's there.

Frequently, we want to know what someone else would think of something or what they would do in a particular situation. Without being able to ask them, there's a limit on what we can do. But there is one technique that may give us a pretty good sense of what others think.

Consider the problem of what to talk about when we meet new people. Meeting new people can be daunting, especially for people who are naturally shy. It can be scary not knowing how another person will react to us. It can be a bit daunting not knowing what to talk about with other people.

In his best-selling book, *How to Make Friends and Influence People*, Dale Carnegie provided some guidance on this (Carnegie 1990). Carnegie, born in 1888, had an interesting career, starting as a travelling salesman. He developed ideas, wrote books, and developed courses on self-improvement, salesmanship, public speaking, and interpersonal skills. He realized that we present ourselves in many different social situations. Through books and lectures, he gave people practical advice on how to manage presentation encounters.

Carnegie figured out what one should talk about with other people if one wants to be perceived as a great conversationalist. He figured this out using the golden rule. He asked, "What is it that I like to talk about?" The answer was himself. He realized that most people would rather talk about their own lives than to listen to someone else go on about theirs. To be a great conversationalist, Carnegie advised, all one had to do was to ask some questions, listen to the answers, and let other people talk about their favorite topic. Carnegie found that one doesn't really need to say much at all to be a great conversationalist. One just needs to be a good listener.

When you don't know what's in someone's head, you might start by asking yourself, "What would I be thinking in a similar circumstance?" I was confronted with this type of problem in my care of psoriasis patients. Many people with psoriasis on their skin, perhaps a third of them, also have psoriasis in their joints, a condition called psoriatic arthritis. Dermatologists are trained to recognize and treat psoriasis skin lesions. The diagnosis of psoriasis can usually be made from across the room. Dermatologists know about a host of different treatments for the skin lesions. Faced with a patient with very complicated psoriasis, even who has failed multiple treatments in the past, dermatologists can offer hope and new approaches. But when a patient with psoriasis says, "Doc, my joints are hurting," dermatologists may be at a bit of a loss.

As good as I am at managing psoriasis, I'm not a rheumatologist, a specialist in the diagnosis and management of joint disease. I'm not familiar with detailed examination of muscles and joints. I can't evaluate x-rays of joints; I wouldn't even know what kind of x-rays to order. And psoriatic arthritis isn't the only kind of joint problem a patient with psoriasis could have; while I assume most psoriasis patients with joint pain have psoriatic arthritis, I don't have the skills to reliably tell what form of arthritis they have or how that might affect the treatment they need. I am familiar with a number of treatments for psoriasis skin lesions that also help psoriatic arthritis, but I wouldn't know for sure if the joints are adequately controlled—and that scares me because psoriatic arthritis can cause permanent joint damage.

As someone who regularly sees psoriasis patients, I frequently see patients who have psoriatic arthritis. I need to know what I should do for these patients, and I can find out by asking an expert, a joint specialist, a rheumatologist. Before meeting with them, though, I don't know what advice they would offer. We can predict what advice a rheumatologist would give about managing psoriatic arthritis by using Carnegie's golden rule.

While a dermatologist doesn't know what rheumatologists would say a dermatologist should do if he or she saw a patient with joint disease, dermatologists know exactly what they would want rheumatologists to do if they saw a patient with skin disease. If a rheumatologist were to see a patient for psoriatic arthritis who also had psoriasis skin lesions, we would advise them, "First, do a complete skin exam to assess the extent of the skin problem. If the skin lesions are a minor problem that doesn't bother the patient much, it's OK to give the patient a topical cortisone to use when the need arises. If the patient has really bad psoriasis that needs more than topical cortisone, refer the patient to me so I can choose the best treatment for them. And if the joints are bad and need a potent medicine that will clear up the patient's skin anyway, go ahead and use it—I'll be glad to see the patient if there are any leftover lesions that need more help."

Based on what dermatologists would want rheumatologists to do about skin lesions, we can use Carnegie's rule to predict what rheumatologists would want dermatologists to do for the joints. "First do a complete muscle and joint exam to evaluate the extent of the problem. If there's no joint destruction and the symptoms aren't particularly bothersome, go ahead and give the patient some ibuprofen (Motrin) or naproxen (Alleve). If that doesn't work, or if the joint disease is more severe than that, please refer them to me so I can choose the best treatment for them. If the skin rash is so bad that it needs potent medication that may fix the arthritis, go ahead and use it. I'll be glad to see the patient if there are joint symptoms that aren't relieved."

It is possible that the culture of rheumatologists is so different from the culture of dermatologists that they would say something completely different. A small survey of rheumatologists from around the world was done to determine how dermatologists should be involved in the management of psoriasis patients with joint disease. Rheumatologists' recommendations for management of the joints in dermatologists' patients with psoriasis were quite similar to dermatologists' recommendations for how rheumatologists should manage skin disease in their patients with psoriatic arthritis.

Had dermatologists considered putting themselves in the patient's shoes, they might have figured out a lot sooner that tachyphylaxis wasn't "the more you use the medicine, the less it worked," but that it was "the less you use the medicine, the less it works." If dermatologists had considered how messy the ointments they were prescribing were and asked themselves, "What would I do if the doctor asked me to put this on twice a day for the rest of my life," they might have thought, *After a while, I'd probably give up and ask for something different. And I probably wouldn't embarrass myself by telling the doctor I had stopped using the medication.*

When people are in another compartment, we may not know what they are thinking. But as a first approximation, we can follow Carnegie's golden rule and assume that other people tend to think very much like we do. Often (as we'll see) it doesn't seem that way, but we're all wired the same way, and our similarities are usually far greater than our differences. When we're trying to figure out how others would view things, we ought to think about how we would view things if we were in their shoes. In chemistry or physics, we'd call this symmetry. It is remarkable how this simple, golden rule-like approach accurately predicts human responses. It is also remarkable how considering other people's viewpoints helps understand problems and conflicts we see around us. We are not as different from others as we often think we are.

Part 2

Things We See That
Are Not Representative

You Can Be Wrong When You Trust What You Do See

There are things in the world that we just don't see. We have to be careful about drawing conclusions about them. Dermatologists made the mistake of thinking tachyphylaxis is *the more you use the medicine the less it works* because they were making assumptions about something they couldn't see. Dermatologists were assuming patients were using their medications when they weren't.

Most of the time, though, we draw conclusions about things we do see. We make direct observations of events all the time. These observations allow us to draw conclusions with confidence. When we observe things often enough, we're not just confident, we draw conclusions about them with assurance. Some things are just obvious. The word "obvious" comes from a Latin root that means "to be in the way." "Obvious" refers to things that are easily seen and, therefore, easily understood. The problem is that in many cases these "obvious" conclusions, though they are easily seen, are wrong. Even though we have direct observations to draw upon, the compartments into which we are organized can cause the brightest, best trained, and most caring people to make judgments that are completely and utterly wrong.

I specialize in the management of patients with psoriasis. One of the best treatments for psoriasis is ultraviolet light treatment. Sun exposure helps most people with psoriasis. In fact, there's a lot more psoriasis in Michigan than in Florida. There's even a specialized psoriasis treatment center at the Dead Sea in Israel where bathing and sun exposure can help clear psoriasis. But getting sun exposure on a regular basis or traveling to Israel isn't practical for most people. Many dermatologists have an ultraviolet light box in their office so they can give patients ultraviolet light treatments. Unfortunately, coming to the office three or more times a week for the treatments can be terribly inconvenient too.

While lecturing to a group of dermatologists, I mentioned that if patients with psoriasis can't come to the office for ultraviolet light treatments, they could get a home ultraviolet light box, or they could try a tanning bed. While tanning beds don't have the same kind of ultraviolet light that we have in the office (and they aren't regulated or monitored the way dermatologists' light units are), tanning beds do work for many people with psoriasis. One of the dermatologists in the audience became agitated upon hearing the suggestion that tanning beds could be used for psoriasis. First, dermatologists hate tanning beds. The idea of sending anyone to a tanning bed is anathema to many dermatologists. More importantly, though, this particular dermatologist *knew* that tanning beds don't help psoriasis, and he didn't mind telling me so in front of everyone at the lecture. "Feldman," he said, "you've gone too far. I've listened patiently to some of these wild ideas you have. But this is simply wrong. Tanning beds do not work for psoriasis! I've seen patient after patient who tried tanning, and none of them cleared up. Tanning beds put out ultraviolet A light, not ultraviolet B. UVB is effective. UVA isn't. If you want psoriasis patients to get better with light treatments, you have to give them light treatment in the office."

While tanning beds may not be the first choice of treatment for psoriasis, they are an effective treatment for many patients. Many of the psoriasis patients I have sent to a tanning bed have improved. The ultraviolet light at the Dead Sea Psoriasis Treatment Center is primarily ultraviolet A light. Two well-done research studies published in top dermatology journals have shown that tanning bed treatments are effective for psoriasis (Carlin 2003; Fleischer 1997). Why did this dermatologist think tanning beds didn't work for psoriasis? Let's consider his experience with ultraviolet light treatments for psoriasis.

First, the phototherapy he offers in his office is a very effective psoriasis treatment. This excellent dermatologist, one who specializes in psoriasis and light treatment, would treat many psoriasis patients with his light unit and would see them improve. Assume for a moment that ultraviolet light treatment in his office clears the disease in 80 percent of patients with psoriasis. If he treated ten patients with his ultraviolet light unit, the psoriasis would clear up in eight of them.

Using an indoor tanning bed may or may not be quite as effective as ultraviolet light treatments given in the doctor's office, but let's just assume for a moment that tanning were just as effective as office-based light treatment, that it would also clear 80 percent of the people who tried it.[2] If this dermatologist who doesn't recommend tanning sees ten people who came in after trying a tanning bed for psoriasis, how many of them would be clear? Well, tanning is 80 percent effective, and he saw ten people who tried it, so this shouldn't be a very difficult math problem. Many people would say eight, thinking that if he saw ten people who tried the

---

[2.] This is just a hypothetical thought experiment. We don't know the exact percentage of people who clear with tanning for psoriasis, but, as you'll see, that is of little importance.

tanning bed, then eight would be clear. But that's not exactly what would happen, at least not from the view of this dermatologist. Anyone who tried tanning for their psoriasis and cleared up would not come see this dermatologist for their psoriasis. Since the tanning cleared up the skin lesions, the skin is clear, and the patient wouldn't need to come in. If this dermatologist saw ten people who tried tanning, they would be ten people who didn't clear! Relying on his observations, this dermatologist wouldn't *think* tanning didn't work; he would *know* tanning didn't work. He would say with assurance, "I've seen patient after patient who tried tanning, and none of them cleared up." From his experience, he got a very wrong sense of the actual efficacy of tanning for psoriasis.

I've misjudged treatments myself, and one time the mistake was of royal proportions. There are some new drugs for psoriasis called tumor necrosis factor inhibitors. These are high-tech, bioengineered drugs whose development was based on advances in our understanding of the immune system. Psoriasis is caused by an overactive immune system, and tumor necrosis factor—we'll call it TNF—plays an important role in the process. The new TNF inhibitors block the effect of TNF in the skin and are very effective for controlling psoriasis and related immune diseases. You may have seen TV commercials for a couple of these drugs, Enbrel and Humira. These new drugs are very expensive, but they are more effective and considerably safer than some of our older psoriasis treatments (Cordoro 2007).

For the patients who need them, for example when psoriasis doesn't get better with ultraviolet light treatments, TNF inhibitors can be life-changing medications. One patient with horrible psoriasis came to see me. The psoriasis also affected his joints. The patient, a man in his thirties, had young children, and the psoriasis and arthritis were so debilitating that he had trouble playing soccer or doing other physical activities with his children.

The extensive inflammation in his body made him feel weak and tired. He had tried many traditional psoriasis and psoriatic arthritis treatments. None of them helped.

I prescribed etanercept for him. Etanercept, also called Enbrel, is a TNF inhibitor. At the time the young man with the severe psoriasis came to see me, etanercept had been recently approved by the Food and Drug Administration as a treatment for psoriasis and psoriatic arthritis. After the first dose of the medication, the young man started to feel better. After the first week, he noticed dramatic improvement in his joint pains and could see that his skin was getting better. His energy level began to improve too. In fact, he didn't even realize how badly the psoriasis had been affecting him until the etanercept cleared up the psoriasis and the psoriatic arthritis. It was like a great fog had lifted. He was now out on the fields playing soccer with his children, something he couldn't do before. His entire attitude about life had improved.

TNF inhibitors are great! But the benefit comes at a cost. There was a lot of money invested in the development and marketing of etanercept. The drug costs nearly $20,000 a year for a single patient. That kind of money can affect the manufacturer's bottom line and stock price. As TNF inhibitors were being developed, before the Food and Drug Administration approval, investment bankers wanted information on how well these drugs would work for psoriasis. Etanercept and another TNF inhibitor called infliximab were already approved and used for patients with rheumatoid arthritis. But that market was somewhat limited. There are 6 million people with psoriasis in the United States. Many of them have severe psoriasis that wasn't well controlled with the older, more traditional treatments. Do the math. At $20,000 per patient per year, investment bankers were calculating that if TNF inhibitors were helpful for psoriasis too, they could be even bigger blockbuster drugs.

Before TNF drugs had been approved for psoriasis, before I began prescribing them in my practice, my phone would ring regularly with calls from investment bankers wondering if TNF inhibitors helped psoriasis. At the time, I told them I thought it was very doubtful that TNF inhibitors would do much good for psoriasis. There was one published study on a small group of psoriasis patients who had received infliximab. The drug seemed to work *better than any other psoriasis drug ever tested.* But to me, that seemed like a fluke. "The drug would not work nearly that well if a larger, better study had been done," I told the bankers.

The investment bankers asked how I knew. They asked if I had experience using TNF inhibitors for my psoriasis patients. I told them I had not, but that I had patients with psoriasis who had tried TNF inhibitors. These were patients who had psoriatic arthritis and psoriasis. They had seen rheumatologists for their joints and had been given TNF inhibitors as a treatment for the arthritis. I confidently told the investment bankers that not one of the patients seeing me for psoriasis had clearing of their skin with the TNF inhibitor prescribed by a rheumatologist for psoriatic arthritis.

There's now an enormous body of research showing that etanercept, infliximab, and other TNF inhibitors are very, very effective treatments for severe psoriasis. Larger studies were done with infliximab, and the drug proved to be *even more effective* than it was in the initial small trial. Many patients with even the most severe forms of the disease may clear up very rapidly with TNF treatment. TNF inhibitors have been life-altering drugs for hundreds of thousands of people with psoriasis. I have since treated many patients with these drugs, and the great majority are much improved using them. So why didn't TNF inhibitors clear the rash in any of the first patients I saw who were treated with them? Was I just unlucky?

In retrospect, it is kind of obvious what had happened. When a rheumatologist gave patients a TNF inhibitor for their arthritis, the psoriasis either cleared up or it didn't. Most of the time, the psoriasis did clear up. Once patients' skin lesions disappeared, those patients didn't need advice on treating their skin disease, so they didn't come to see me. Occasionally, a patient treated with a TNF inhibitor for their arthritis would not have much improvement in their skin disease. Those patients did come to see me. It didn't matter how well the TNF inhibitors worked for the skin. They might be the most effective psoriasis treatments ever invented. Still, when the TNF inhibitor was prescribed by the joint doctor, I only got to see patients in whom it didn't work.

This phenomenon is a kind of selection bias. Selection bias happens whenever one doesn't get a balanced sample. But what happened in the examples above is a special form of selection bias, a very powerful form of the bias. This kind of selection bias occurs when the reason we observe something is *because it is different from what usually happens*. This kind of selection bias is also very, very common when we are looking at things in a compartment other than our own. If we look at the results of a treatment that was prescribed in a different "compartment" than our own, we commonly don't get a representative picture of the results. We would make a conclusion that would seem obvious, yet it would be wrong.

There are many examples of this bias in dermatology. A seventeen-year-old boy named Jorge came to my office complaining of acne. He had red bumps and small cysts on his face and upper back. He had already tried a widely promoted treatment for acne called Proactiv (Proactiv 2007). Proactiv is a popular product. There are TV and radio commercials for it and print ads too. Famous celebrities promote the product. Advertisements for Proactiv may show striking before—and after-treatment photographs. Perhaps more people use Proactiv as an acne treatment than any other single product. But for Jorge, Proactiv didn't work very well at all. In my experience, that is typical. Seeing acne patients is the bread and butter of dermatology practice, and we frequently see patients who've tried Proactiv for their acne. Yet personally, I don't think I've seen a single acne patient who tried Proactiv and found that it adequately controlled their acne. I'm not just saying I haven't seen Proactiv completely clear up acne. In my acne patient population, the patients who tried Proactiv not only found that their face didn't clear up completely; it didn't even improve enough that they were happy with the result.

Of course, my experience isn't particularly helpful for knowing how effective Proactiv is. I don't know if Proactiv improves acne in 1 percent of people who use it or if it completely clears acne up in 99.9 percent of people who use it. I do know, however, if Jorge had seen the ad for Proactiv on TV, tried the product, and was happy with the result, he probably wouldn't have come to my office for acne treatment. No matter how effective Proactiv is, I'll probably never see a patient for acne that cleared up with Proactiv. There's just no reason for such patients to see me if their acne is already gone.

A child visited my office with warts on her hands. We don't have very good treatments for warts. The most common treatment used by dermatologists is to freeze the warts with liquid nitrogen. The freezing and thawing process kills the skin, just as a burn would. Freezing the skin can be painful, and it doesn't always work to get rid of the wart. The freezing and thawing process doesn't kill the virus that causes warts. Freezing just kills the skin where the virus is. Hopefully, when the dead skin falls off, it takes the virus with it. Sometimes it does; sometimes it doesn't.

The mother of the child with warts had heard about a wart treatment that could be done at home. It was also a freeze product, a spray that could be bought without a prescription in pharmacies. The over-the-counter spray product doesn't contain liquid nitrogen and isn't as cold as the medication we dermatologists use to treat warts. The mom wanted to know if the product was effective. I told the mom that I've seen many children with warts and that some of them had tried the over-the-counter freeze product. Not a single one of them had cleared up their warts with the over-the-counter product. Not one. In my experience, the over-the-counter product had never cleared anybody's warts. Some dermatologists might conclude that the colder temperature of liquid nitrogen makes it more effective than the over-the-counter spray for wart treatment. Some dermatologists might wonder why the Food and Drug Administration allows a company to market an ineffective treatment. I explained to the mom that my experience of the effectiveness of the over-the-counter product might not be a very good way to assess the effectiveness of the product. Anyone whose warts clear up with the over-the-counter freeze spray would not be likely to come to my office asking for help for their warts.

When we observe something *because it is different from what usually happens,* we can get a very warped view of reality. It is important to be on the lookout for this kind of selection bias. Often we are very confident about what we know when it is based on our firsthand experiences. Those experiences can be misleading, sometimes very misleading.

Do Primary Care Doctors Know Anything About Skin Disease?

Selection bias can have dramatic effects on the way people view each other as exemplified by dermatologists' experiences with primary care doctors. The early 1990s was a scary time for dermatologists. Some people wondered if dermatologists would soon be driving taxis (Stern 1986). Gatekeeping managed care was a growing phenomenon, and dermatologists feared for themselves and for their patients. Primary care doctors were getting paid more when they referred less. People knew that primary care doctors weren't going to start doing neurosurgery, but there was a real sense that primary care providers might handle the treatment of skin diseases without the need for dermatologists.

Some dermatologists knew that the shift of skin disease management from dermatologists to primary care doctors wouldn't last. There was no way primary care doctors would be able to adequately manage patients with skin disease. How did dermatologists know? It was kind of obvious, actually. Dermatologists knew from experience that primary care doctors couldn't handle skin disease problems. Dermatologists were certain of it.

A typical dermatologist might see twenty or thirty patients a day, sometimes more. Most of these patients had already been to their primary care doctor for their skin problem. They went to their primary care physician first. In a typical day, not one of these patients would come in with skin disease that had been effectively managed by the patient's primary care doctor. Not one! It wasn't just that 25 percent or even 50 percent of these patients who had seen the primary care doctor first about their skin disease had not been successfully treated. Not 75 percent or even 90 percent. On a typical day in the dermatologist's office, none of the patients who had already seen a primary care doctor for their condition had been effectively treated.

Consider the typical dermatologist's experience. If just ten of the dermatologist's patients a day were referred from primary care, and the dermatologist saw patients just 200 days a year, that's 2,000 patients referred from primary care each year. The number of those 2,000 that the primary care doctors managed to treat successfully could be counted on just one hand. And that's a conservative estimate. Most dermatologists probably see many more than 2,000 patients a year and still less than a handful of those patients come with a skin disease that the primary care doctor managed to control.

Based on that experience, dermatologists knew they were needed. They knew that they wouldn't be replaced by primary care doctors. To dermatologists, it seemed that primary care physicians knew very little about skin disease. Dermatologists saw patients with skin disease that primary care doctors either couldn't diagnose or misdiagnosed. Dermatologists saw patients who got inadequate treatment or, not so infrequently, treatment that actually made things worse!

There were patients with fungus infections of the skin—athlete's foot or jock itch—misdiagnosed as having an allergic dermatitis. These patients had often been treated by the family doctor with cortisone medicines that made the problem worse. Other patients actually did have allergic dermatitis and had been treated with antifungal medications. Even the most common conditions, like acne, never seemed to improve under the care of the family doctor. The family doctors seemed to have no clue how to accurately diagnose and treat psoriasis. Dermatologists almost never saw anyone for a skin disease that the primary care doctor accurately diagnosed and effectively treated. At the time, it seemed primary care doctors couldn't get anyone's skin disease cleared up.

Part of my research career was spent studying this phenomenon. We studied the kinds of skin conditions primary care doctors were seeing. They tended to be run-of-the-mill skin disease problems. We looked at training differences and reviewed the literature on differences between primary care doctors' and dermatologists' ability to recognize different skin diseases from photographs. Using national databases, my colleague Alan Fleischer and I analyzed the differences between the care provided by dermatologists and by primary care physicians. There were some important differences. There were also a lot of similarities. Our work was well funded and even led to awards from the American Academy of Dermatology.

But there was one little hitch. If a patient saw their primary care physician, was accurately diagnosed and was given a treatment that cleared up their rash, they would not have been very likely to see a dermatologist for that rash! People whose skin condition was cured by the family doctor were cured; once cured, they didn't go to the dermatologist. For all we knew, primary care doctors were actually clearing up skin diseases in most of their patients. If primary care doctors cleared the skin problem in 99 percent of their patients, dermatologists only got to see the other

1 percent. Because dermatologists practice in one compartment and family doctors in another, dermatologists' impressions of family physicians were profoundly distorted.

Experience is not always a good teacher. Dermatologists based their impressions of the quality of dermatologic care offered by family doctors on dermatologists' experiences. These impressions did not provide a representative sample of the care family doctors provide. Dermatologists' experiences were terribly biased, as commonly happens when people in one compartment use their experience to judge people in another compartment.

Doctors' Impressions
of Other Doctors

The kind of bias that affects dermatologists' impressions of treatment affects their impression of other physicians. One might think that doctors have a good understanding of the medical care offered by other doctors. But bias has dramatic impact on the ways doctors in different specialties view each other. Although all doctors start as medical students in school together, they eventually separate into different specialty group compartments. This compartmentalization colors how different specialties view each other.

We considered the example of dermatology and primary care. How many dermatologists in the United States have ever seen a patient for a skin disease that had been effectively managed by the patient's family physician? None. No dermatologist has ever seen that, and no dermatologist ever would. Only treatment failures are referred to a dermatologist, a simple fact that makes it too easy for us to believe that family physicians do not effectively manage their skin disease patients.

This kind of bias also affects how other specialties view dermatologists. One of the most common problems dermatologists treat is skin cancer. There are several types of skin cancer. The most serious of these is melanoma. Melanoma is a cancer of the pigment cells in the skin. If not caught early, it can spread through the body. Fortunately, melanoma is much less common than the other main types of skin cancer. The other two main types of skin cancer are basal cell carcinoma and squamous cell carcinoma. While these types of skin cancers are very common, fortunately they can be treated very easily. They can be cut out. Some can even be removed by scraping them off. But some basal cell and squamous cell skin cancers are more problematic. In certain areas of the face, they tend to invade deeply. Some grow with a pattern of little fingers that spread through the adjacent skin. The traditional ways of removing skin cancer don't work particularly well for these more aggressive forms of the disease. Squamous cell carcinoma is a bit worse than basal cell carcinoma because squamous cell carcinoma can spread to other places in the body—it can metastasize—though not as often as do melanomas.

Some dermatologists do a special kind of surgery for more aggressive basal cell and squamous cell skin cancers, a procedure called Mohs micrographic surgery. Pioneered by Dr. Fredrick Mohs, in this type of surgery, the dermatologist carefully checks the edges of the tumor being removed to make sure the tumor is completely eliminated. While other forms of skin cancer removal may be 90 to 95 percent effective, micrographic surgery is close to 100 percent effective at completely removing the cancer from the skin.

The goal of skin cancer treatment is to get the tumor out before it has a chance to metastasize. Once the skin cancer spreads, removing the skin tumor is like closing the barn door after the cows have left. Micrographic surgery doesn't treat metastases. Fortunately, these metastases are rare events because people usually get checked and have the skin cancer removed before the tumor spreads internally.

Dermatologists aren't the only doctors that care for patients with skin cancer. Ear, nose, and throat specialists (the technical term for these doctors is otolaryngologists) also see patients with skin cancer. Typically, they don't do micrographic surgery. They tend to just cut the cancer out with a margin of normal skin around the lesion. Otolaryngologists are also the doctors that operate on lymph nodes of the head and neck should a tumor have spread internally to those nodes.

Otolaryngologists may see that 9 out of 10 squamous cell carcinomas they excise are cured. But when otolaryngologists see a patient who had a squamous cell carcinoma treated by a dermatologist who used micrographic surgery, it is almost surely because that tumor metastasized to regional nodes. Even if micrographic surgery done by a dermatologist cures 999 out of 1,000 tumors, the otolaryngologist will see in referral only the 1 in 1,000 that metastasized before the primary tumor was removed. There's usually no reason for the otolaryngologist to see any of the other 999 whose cancer was fully removed. In the experience of some otolaryngologists, every time they saw a patient who had micrographic surgery for a squamous cell carcinoma, the carcinoma metastasized. Based on such observations, some otolaryngologists have been misled to believe that Mohs micrographic surgery—the most effective form of surgery for nonmelanoma skin cancer—*causes* squamous cell carcinomas to metastasize.

One can see how surgeons could get a warped view of the care that dermatologists provide. If each specialty only sees the others' failures, they end up thinking less of each other. Some dermatologists do various cosmetic surgery procedures; it's not likely that many of the patients happy with the result are going to go to a plastic surgeon to brag about the care provided by the dermatologist. More likely, the dermatologist's successes will stay with the dermatology practice, and only patients dissatisfied with the surgical outcome will see a plastic surgeon. The plastic surgeon will be left with a very poor impression of the care offered by the dermatologist. The same holds true for the plastic surgeon's patient and the dermatologist. Even within a specialty, one doctor is much more likely to see a colleague's failures than their successes.

This type of bias affects perceptions between many different groups of health care providers. There is controversy about what roles physician extenders—physician assistants and nurse practitioners—should play in providing medical care to the public. Some doctors feel very strongly that patients with illnesses should see a doctor, not a physician extender. Doctors who feel this way do so not because they are concerned about their livelihoods (though it is easy to think that's the reason they feel this way). Doctors who feel this way are concerned about patient welfare. These doctors don't think patients should have to see what the doctor believes is a lesser-quality health care provider. It is easy to see how physicians who have never worked with a physician extender could think that physician extenders offer lesser quality of care. The doctor who hasn't worked with a physician assistant or nurse practitioner will have seen only their failures, never their successes.

People often misjudge other people's thinking. Because we can't see into other people's heads, we have to be very careful when drawing conclusions about other people's motivations. When a physician assistant or nurse practitioner hears a doctor say, "Patients should see doctors. Physician assistants and nurse practitioners don't offer good medical care," the physician assistant or nurse practitioner probably thinks that that doctor is a greedy person who only cares about protecting his or her turf, not about patients' well-being. On the contrary, the doctors who say this sort of thing care deeply about patients. In fact, *the most caring* doctors may be *the most passionate and vociferous* in their opposition to physician extenders. These doctors are basing their concerns on their experiences. Their experiences tell them that physician extenders offer inadequate medical care. These experiences are *extraordinarily biased and erroneous*, but the doctor doesn't know that. Physician extenders give patients great medical care, but the doctor who doesn't work with a physician extender doesn't see any of the patients who were treated successfully.

Making sure patients get great medical care is an emotionally powerful issue for doctors. Doctors spend years and years in study so they can give patients the best possible medical care. Doctors don't believe patients should settle for less. So it isn't easy to convince doctors who have only seen bad outcomes from physician extenders that extenders are actually doing a good job. Doctors care deeply about their patients, and these doctors' experiences tell them that physician assistants don't do a good job. In the political discussions among physicians about the roles of physician assistants and nurse practitioners, doctors who haven't worked with a physician assistant or nurse practitioner need to be a bit circumspect about their experience.

These doctors need to realize their experience, even if it is extensive, may be incomplete and sometimes even completely inaccurate. Seeing past the bias is difficult enough when a neutral issue is at hand. When the issue is tied to strong emotions and when the bias reinforces preconceived notions, it is very difficult to see beyond what seems obvious. Sometimes, the brightest and most caring people are at the center of conflicts that have resulted from misperceptions due to compartments.

Surveying Patients' Impressions of Doctors

Selection bias doesn't just affect doctors' perceptions of other doctors. Selection bias can also affect the public's perception of doctors and many other issues. I've done informal surveys of patients' and doctors' impressions of how satisfied patients are with their doctors. I asked people to tell me—on a scale of 0 to 10—how satisfied they think patients are with their doctors. Both doctors and nondoctors gave me a range of answers, most in the range of 4-6. A couple of doctors thought most patients give their doctor the benefit of the doubt and that the average score would be more like 8.

How satisfied are patients with their doctor? Well, to hear politicians talk about health care, you'd think people would be pretty unhappy. The news frequently reports problems with our health care system. The doctors I surveyed didn't seem particularly enthusiastic about high levels of patient satisfaction.

What are patients' impressions of their doctors? The National Psoriasis Foundation wanted to find out. The foundation is dedicated to improving the lives of people with psoriasis through education and advocacy, promoting access to good treatment, and working to find a cure for the condition. The foundation was started on August 29, 1966, the 30th birthday of Beverly Foster, a Portland, Oregon, resident who suffered from severe psoriasis. On that day, Beverly's husband placed a tiny classified advertisement in a Portland newspaper, asking people with psoriasis to call Beverly so she could talk with someone who understood what she was going through. The Psoriasis Foundation, now thirty-five years old, was led for twenty-eight of those years by former CEO Gail Zimmerman. Under Gail's leadership, the foundation grew to encompass tens of thousands of members, and it started an ambitious Gene Bank project to help researchers better understand the cause of psoriasis so that a cure could be found. The foundation also worked to help educate doctors about psoriasis. That's how my affiliation with the foundation began, as a young dermatologist who knew very little about psoriasis but who wanted to learn more so I could provide better care for my patients.

Gail recounted to me that for many years the situation facing patients appeared grim. There seemed to be no good dermatologists to help them. "Patient after patient would call our office complaining that they couldn't find a good doctor. There were new treatments for psoriasis, but what good were they if patients couldn't find a good doctor to prescribe them? The foundation was able to meet patients' needs for education, but we were unable to help people find a good doctor. Listening to so many people complain and not being able to do a thing about it was frustrating and depressing for us.

"In 1985, we decided to do a formal survey of our members to better understand and document the problem patients were having. We surveyed 10,000 members" (Zimmerman 2007).

Many of those surveyed reported that they wanted their doctors to be more understanding, but overall, they were very happy with their doctors. Gail was perplexed. It didn't make sense. People would call into the foundation complaining and complaining, but the survey showed that the vast majority of members were actually happy with their dermatologists. The survey apparently was not a very good assessment of the problem as Gail knew from all the calls she received that patients weren't as happy as the survey showed.

In 2001, the Psoriasis Foundation did a second survey. This time, the Psoriasis Foundation decided to make the survey more scientific. They enlisted the help of several dermatologists who specialized in epidemiology, the study of factors affecting the health and illness of populations. Dr. Robert Stern, professor of dermatology at Harvard Medical School and vice chairman of dermatology of the Beth Israel Deaconess Medical Center in Boston, dermatology's leader in the discipline of epidemiology, led the research team. In developing the survey, the team identified available measures that were the most scientifically rigorous. Then, working with a commercial survey research firm, they developed a methodology to get an accurate assessment of patients' quality of life and concerns about their disease.

The results of the survey surprised Gail and her staff at the Psoriasis Foundation. "The survey found that many patients would have liked to be treated with more aggressive treatment. Overall, however, they reported being very happy with their dermatologists. Psoriasis Foundation members loved their doctors," she said. The National Psoriasis Foundation staff was dumbfounded. The survey findings were just the opposite of what they were expecting. How could it be that their members were so happy, yet all the calls and letters they received were complaints? Gail says, "The foundation was continually getting calls from patients who were unhappy, who said they were on their tenth dermatologist and couldn't find a good one. It seemed like nobody liked their doctor." The second survey had been done in the most scientifically compelling manner.

—

It took awhile, but the foundation realized that most of their members really were very happy with their doctors. The foundation staff had been misled because none of the happy patients called or wrote out of frustration when they had a doctor they liked. Only dissatisfied patients did that.

It is pretty easy in the Internet age to gauge people's satisfaction with their doctors. I started an online patient satisfaction survey, *www.DrScore.com*, that lets patients freely rate doctors and lets the public look up doctor ratings. Tens of thousands of people have used the site to rate their doctors. It takes just a few minutes, and it is a great way to help doctors get feedback on how they are doing. While there isn't enough data in the system to score all doctors yet (you can visit www.DrScore.com if you want to add ratings of your doctors), an analysis was done of doctors who did have twenty or more ratings to see how satisfied patients tend to be. The average doctor had a patient satisfaction score of 9.3 out of 10!

My gerontologist sent me for a colonoscopy. It was a remarkably good medical service experience. The gastroenterologist sent me detailed instructions concerning the procedure. The instructions were clear and unambiguous. They described my responsibilities—the preprocedure preparation (what products to purchase, how to take them, and what I was to expect when I did), the need to bring someone with me to the procedure to drive me home, and what to do to relieve discomfort after the procedure. When I presented for the procedure, I was greeted quickly and warmly by the reception desk. Current magazines and a television were there to help shorten the wait. They weren't needed, as shortly after I sat down, the nursing staff took me back to the preparation area. They attended to my privacy and told me what to expect. I was taken to the procedure room where I was given drugs that have prevented me from remembering anything about the actual procedure. After the procedure, I was given detailed written postprocedure instructions and sent home with my wife. The whole experience, from beginning to end, was perfect. It was a perfect 10.

I didn't read about my colonoscopy experience in the newspaper. There was no coverage of it on television or radio news programs. There wasn't even an Internet blog about it, nor was there YouTube coverage of the event. This episode of wonderful medical care was completely invisible to the public as though it had never happened. The experiences of all the other patients whose procedures went well that day are equally invisible. However, had something really bad happened, had I died as a result of the procedure, it would have been news. It would have been the kind of exceptional event that would make the daily paper. The worse I had suffered, the more newsworthy it would have been.

Doctors are completely dedicated to their patients. They spend years upon years to prepare to be doctors, to make sure they give patients great medical care. Yet even doctors don't know how well doctors are doing. Doctors read the news, they see the TV, or listen to the radio. They learn of dissatisfaction with medical care. Doctors see other doctors' patients, often because the patient wasn't entirely satisfied with the results of the first doctor's care. It shouldn't be surprising that people's *sense* of patient satisfaction is so much lower than patient satisfaction actually is. People know they are satisfied with their own doctor, but they can't see what's in other people's minds. We see what is reported in the news, but the news rarely reports when a patient has had a great medical experience, even rarer, a satisfying one. These are routine. They are the norm. They aren't news.

Every day we have experiences that tell us about the world around us. Many times, we get a warped impression of what's going on. For example, if someone has liposuction and everything goes well, we're not likely to hear about it. It's unlikely to make the newspaper and would certainly not be a cover story. Yet if the person having liposuction dies from the procedure, we probably would hear about it. It would be news. It might make the front page of the newspaper or, if the situation were bad enough, it might garner national attention. In fact, though this kind of horrible event rarely occurs with liposuction, the only time we might hear about liposuction is that rare occasion. If we aren't actually doing liposuction or seeing a representative sample of people who do, we might think from our experience that liposuction commonly ends up causing severe problems.

This type of bias has dramatic effects on the way people view the world. It affects how people view other people. Psoriasis patients loved their doctors, but you couldn't tell that from the complaint calls people make to the Psoriasis Foundation. If you want to understand the quality of medical care in the United States—or if you wanted to understand anything else—you don't want to judge it solely on the events that newspapers or TV report! You need to get and assess a more representative sample.

Lee Garrity, City Manager

Selection bias isn't limited to the health care system. Selection bias is exceedingly common when we look at any news. Consider my neighbor, Lee Garrity. Lee is a great neighbor. He's very personable, always cheery and friendly. He's involved in the community, serving on the Goodwill Industries Board of Directors, a Redevelopment Advisory Board, and the Winston-Salem State University Adult Services Advisory Board. Lee once invited me to speak at an evening get-together of his men's group at one of the neighborhood churches. His wife is a homemaker and part-time artist. Some of her work decorates their home. They have two wonderful daughters who enjoy horseback riding. As Lee's neighbor, one thing I know very well about him is that he does a great job keeping up his yard.

Lee is also the city manager of Winston-Salem (City of Winston-Salem 2007). Winston-Salem is a town of about 200,000 people. As city manager, Lee is responsible for sanitation, water and sewer services, waste disposal, storm water, and cemeteries. He's also responsible for the police and fire departments as well as emergency management. And he's responsible for our streets, our transit authority, and our parking. And he takes care of community and economic development and a variety of leisure services (including parks, recreation centers, a sports complex, and a convention center), not to mention overseeing city government purchasing, employees, policy, and finances.

Lee oversees a staff of 2,500 people. He manages a budget of about $400 million, which is more than the gross domestic product of some countries. He does a fabulous job too. Winston-Salem is a wonderful place to live. We have clean water to drink, good roads to drive on, and a safe environment in which to bring up our children. The downtown is becoming a great place to go for visiting art galleries or dining. There's wireless Internet service downtown too. We take our children to play in the city parks in spring and to city pools in summer. Our neighborhood is full of mature oak trees, which give us very nice shade but which drop an inordinate number of leaves come fall. It's no problem, though, as we just rake the leaves to the street, and the city picks them up.

On a typical day in Winston-Salem, all 2,500 people working for Lee do their jobs and do them well. But a few times a year, something else happens. Maybe only 2,499 people did their jobs well, or maybe something happened that none of the 2,500 people could control. When that happens, Lee Garrity gets covered in our town paper, usually on the front page.

When 2,499 of the 2,500 city employees do their job exceptionally well, do we notice them? No, we don't. Do we notice the one who doesn't? You bet we do, and people complain to Lee when it happens. Except for the day he was named city manager, I don't think Lee has ever made it into our newspaper on any of the many days that everything went right. Why would he? When everything goes the way it is supposed to go, it isn't news. While Lee makes the front page of the local newspaper every now and then, it isn't because all 2,500 people he supervises did a great job that day.

If you were to use only what's reported in the news as a way of evaluating Lee's performance as city manager, you'd say he can't do anything right. Nearly every time you see his name, it's associated with something bad that has happened. But the reality is that 99.99% of the time, everything Lee is associated with actually goes very well.

Newspapers and TV report news. They tend to do it very well. In reporting the news, newspapers and other news media may interpret the news one way or another, but by and large, day in and day out, they accurately report events that occur. It is big news when they don't (just ask Dan Rather). But just because the newspaper reports events accurately doesn't mean you get a good picture of what's happening in the world. If you use the news to tell you what's going on, you get a warped view of reality. All the ordinary, common things that occur will be invisible; every day, commonplace events are, by definition, not news. News looks for outliers and brings them to our attention. All the unusual events will get reported. The stranger, scarier, and rarer those events are, the more likely they will get covered. Only the truly most unusual events (like the time the White Sox won the World Series) make headlines. Basing our view of the world on what we see in the news is likely to get us into trouble.

"Going Postal"

Selection bias is responsible for much misperception. Sometimes, the degree of misperception is extraordinary. One example of this is related to people's perceptions of the U.S. Postal Service. In 1986, Patrick Henry Sherrill, a Postal Service employee, shot and killed fourteen people at his Oklahoma workplace before turning the gun on himself. In 1991, two former U.S. Postal Service employees, Joseph Harris and Thomas McIlvane, were involved in separate shooting incidents. Harris shot and killed four people including his former boss and two other Postal Service employees in New Jersey. McIlvane killed five people, including himself, in a Michigan post office. Jennifer San Marco, a former employee at a California mail processing plant, shot and killed seven people in 2006, including six postal workers at the facility, before committing suicide (Wikipedia, Going Postal, 2008).

According to Wikipedia, "going postal" is an accepted American English slang term, meaning to suddenly become extremely and uncontrollably angry, possibly violent. The term "going postal" resulted from a series of events in which U.S. Postal Service workers shot and killed managers, fellow workers, and members of the public. Over the eleven-year period from 1986 to 1997, more than forty people were killed in at least twenty incidents involving postal workers. Following this, the term "going postal" began to be applied to murders committed in acts of workplace and nonworkplace rage.

The U.S. Postal Service hates that "going postal" is used in this way. The Postal Service has even sued to stop such use. People like Edmund and Frances Feldman are also offended if they heard someone use the term "going postal" to refer to workplace rage. Ed and Fran are retired United States Postal Service employees. They know a lot about the organization and are proud of the Postal Service and its employees. Ed Feldman would tell you that the Postal Service is the second largest employer in the United States with over 700,000 employees. Ed served in the Postal Service's legal division. His wife Fran served in a variety of capacities, mostly as a writer and editor. When she retired, she was editor of the Postal Inspection Service's journal, a publication that among other things described valiant and successful efforts by postal inspectors to solve crime and apprehend criminals.

Ed and Fran Feldman never killed any of their coworkers, so you've probably never heard of them or the hundreds of thousands of postal workers like them. Unless you are a postal worker yourself, it is not likely you know many of the diligent men and women who process the many millions of pieces of mail that are distributed and delivered across our nation. You may not know any of the over 700,000 employees in the organization, save perhaps your postal carrier or clerks in your neighborhood post office. However, on the rare occasion that a postal worker does become violent, you'd hear about it in the news. When a postal employee does something violent, it *is* news.

Day in and day out, hundreds of thousands of Postal Service employees handle millions of pieces of mail. Tens of billions of letters are handled each year. It is an enormous undertaking. Postal Service employees do this amazing job. They do it well, day in and day out. The phenomenal efficiency of the process and the dedication of the employees isn't something that makes headlines. Delivering all this mail each day is almost a miracle, but at the same time, it has become an ordinary, everyday event. The news doesn't need to report on pieces of mail that arrive promptly and in good condition.

When one of the 700,000 postal workers commits a murder, however, it is news. It is such an extraordinary event it doesn't just make headlines in the city where it occurred. It claims headlines across the country. It is such an attention-generating phenomenon as to have engendered a term, "going postal," in the American English lexicon. In no way, however, are such events indicative of the Postal Service or its employees.

In fact, murder rates among postal employees are quite low, far lower than expected given the number of employees who serve in the U.S. Postal Service. During the eleven-year period from 1986 to 1997 when more than forty people were killed in incidents involving postal workers, the Federal Bureau of Investigation crime statistics report the annual murder rate in the United States ranged from a low of 6.8 to a high of 9.8 per 100,000 people (U.S. Department of Justice 2005). At that rate, one would have expected about sixty murders *per year* among the 700,000 Postal Service employees. The actual rate was fifteen-fold lower!

Using the term "going postal" to refer to workplace rage does a disservice to the U.S. Postal Service and its dedicated employees. "Going postal" should be a synonym for having a steadfast commitment to providing great service and to getting an enormously complex job done well. That the term is used to describe something ugly is indicative of how utterly misleading even accurate news coverage can be.

Other Issues in the Public's View

What we see can be very deceiving. When we look at other groups from a distance, our experiences may be completely useless for understanding that group. Family physicians are good doctors, yet dermatologists never see patients who family doctors cured. Most patients are generally extremely happy with the care they get from their doctors, but people think that overall patient satisfaction is poor. People use the term "going postal" to indicate a state of violent rage, yet your postman is dedicated to giving you great service and is not at all likely to explode in a fit of rage. Our observations may consist of accurate reports of objective facts, yet sometimes reality is completely different from the conclusions we draw from our observations. When we base our conclusions on unarguable, observed facts, it can be very difficult to accept that our conclusions are wrong. We need to keep in mind that the facts we have observed may have been reported because they are extraordinary and completely unrepresentative of what is regular and ordinary.

Perhaps the most important human relations issue of our times involves the United States and our relationship with the Muslim people of the Middle East. Our understanding of Muslims and their understandings of us are affected by the kind of bias that results from newspapers reporting the unusual and not the usual.

Consider what Arab Muslims probably read in their local paper about the United States. Does it make news that each morning Americans lovingly send their children to school? Probably not. Does it make news that Americans go to church to pray for peace? Not likely—that isn't news. The media doesn't report about normal farmers, construction workers, or nurses; there's nothing about people shopping or peacefully visiting their friends and family. The ordinary events that truly characterize our lives or culture are not news.

My neighbor Betsy Brown is a typical American. Betsy, seventy years old, is the oldest of four sisters. She has two children and five grandchildren. Betsy worked as a homemaker and volunteer for twenty years, then worked at the YWCA for another twenty years on programs such as Project New Start, helping female prison inmates and their families get on with their lives. Betsy retired from the Y five years ago. She stays busy doing volunteer work with her husband Walter. Walter, who Betsy says is "a good insurance agent," has his own agency specializing in personal lines insurance. He's now semiretired and likes to spend time golfing. He's an elder in the First Presbyterian Church.

Walter and Betsy tutor once a week at an after-school program for Hispanic children in a former Presbyterian church building that was donated the mission, El Buen Pastor, the good shepherd. Betsy is serving for the second time on the Board of Prodigals Community, a residential substance-abuse recovery program for men and women. Betsy also participates in a weekly Bible study at the local jail and hosts a Bible study for friends at her home once a month. Betsy remains an active participant in church groups, volunteering for service activities for the church and other agencies.

Betsy is like a lot of people who make up the backbone of this great country of ours. Her life is devoted to family, friends, and community. Betsy is a wonderful person, but not extraordinary in the strict sense of the word. The Betsy Browns in America seldom make the front page of our local newspapers and are even less likely to be featured in a story in Middle East newspapers.

What American stories make the Middle East headlines? Instead of reading about Betsy Brown, Arab Muslims probably hear about Britney Spears and Paris Hilton and their "personal issues." They are more likely to read about Enron executives and other crooked businesspeople, not honest insurance agents like Walter Brown. They are probably much more likely to hear about newsmakers such as Congressman Foley and Senator Craig than other legislators. The only American high school they've probably ever heard of is in Columbine. The news doesn't leave them with a very pretty picture of us.

Worse yet, people in the Muslim world hear about every Muslim killed by a U.S.-built F-16 flown by the Israelis; their newspapers probably report the names of the victims and the suffering of the families. Arab Muslims hear about mistreatment of prisoners at Abu Graib, the tens or hundreds of thousands of Iraqis dead and the millions displaced since our invasion, and our support of Israel's invasion of Gaza. If they heard about an American doing something ordinary, like giving to charity or helping in a disaster, they probably dismiss it as atypical of us. I'm not terribly optimistic about the picture they have of us. It almost certainly isn't a picture that is representative of who we truly are. Perhaps some of our movies and TV shows reach some of them. But here's a scary thought: as bad as our movies and TV are at representing our culture, those media probably portray a more accurate assessment of us than the news would. A person might get a better understanding of

Americans by watching *The Simpsons* than they could from reading news covered in an Arab newspaper.

The problem isn't that the Arab media are biased against us. The problem is that even accurate news stories tend to cover that which is out of the ordinary. In the United States, we have access to a broad array of news sources. These sources of information inform our understanding of Arab Muslims. The resulting understanding of Muslims and Islam can be terribly inaccurate. If you pick up a newspaper in most places in the United States and read the word "Muslim" on the front page, the next word is almost certainly "terrorist." If you see the word "Islamic," the next word is probably "fundamentalist," and it probably isn't being used in a complimentary way. In the post-9/11 world, the American media regularly reports on episodes of suicide bombings and other killings in the Middle East; based on those reports, Americans probably get the sense that Islam is a violent religion and that Muslims are violent people.

Given what we see in our news, it's probably hard to believe that the word "Islam" comes from the Arabic word for "submission," referring to submission to G-d's will and the related root word for "peace." There are roughly a billion Muslims in the world. Based on off-the-cuff calculations, the suicide bombers seen in our media probably represent no more than 1/10,000th of 1 percent of all Muslims. If you were to look at a pie chart depicting Muslim people, you would be hard put to see the miniscule slice this represents. Do the terrorists represent typical Muslims? Certainly, they do not. It may be that 99.9999 percent of Muslims are peaceful. Terrorists are no more representative of Muslims than American soldiers or contractors who have committed atrocities against Arab Muslims are representative of Americans. Unfortunately, both get seen in the media, and each affect how Americans and Arab Muslims perceived each another.

To understand Muslims better, we need to look beyond what we see in the news. There are a lot of Betsy Brown-like people in the Muslim world who aren't making our newspapers. We ought to seek out Muslims and talk to them personally. Listening to what the average Christian American thinks Muslims are like is probably a very good source of information for what Christians think of Muslims; it probably isn't a particularly reliable source of information for what Muslims actually are like. One of Betsy Brown's friends passed on advice from a Muslim that you can't establish an understanding relationship with a Muslim "until you've shared a hundred cups with him." This is good advice if we are trying to understand what Muslims are really like.[3]

Despite what we see and hear in the news, the Muslim religion is committed to peaceful, G-d-fearing behavior. The details of the religion don't sound particularly unfamiliar to an American Jew. In many ways, the traditions of Islam are not altogether different from Jewish and Christian traditions. I seek to learn more about Islam from firsthand encounters with Muslims wherever I can, and uniformly they confirm Muslims' devotion to peace.

The notion of peaceful Muslims may seem completely different from what we know of Muslims based on what is published on the cover of our newspapers. We should consider that Muslims probably get completely crazy ideas about how violent our society is (and how violent the Christian religion must be) if they

---

[3.] There are other sources of information that describe facets of Islam that don't make the news. A great resource is The Teaching Company, a company that sells educational lectures on CD/DVD. The Teaching Company offers a wonderful series on Islam and other religions (Teaching Company, 2008). What the course teaches about Islam and Muslims is very different from what little I had learned of Islam and Muslims in my Hebrew School education and from the news media.

draw their conclusions based on what is published about us in their newspapers. We should recognize that the views of both Muslims and Christians of each other may be as biased as some dermatologists' opinions on tanning as a treatment for psoriasis or of the skin disease care offered by family physicians.

We may wonder why there aren't more moderate Muslims speaking out against extremists. It may be that there are many such moderates speaking out, but that they simply aren't as newsworthy as the extremists are. Moreover, we might consider Carnegie's golden rule and wonder if Muslims are asking the same question, "Why aren't there more moderate Christians speaking out against the violence done by the West?"

I had a wonderful conversation with Dr. Samir Hantirah, a Muslim Egyptian dermatologist, at an international psoriasis meeting held in Stockholm, Sweden. There was a break in the meeting for lunch. Box lunches were served. My new acquaintance and I each grabbed a boxed lunch and headed to a bench in a garden outside the meeting building to eat lunch, enjoy Stockholm's beautiful June weather, and learn a little about each other. Dr. Hantirah confirmed that Islam is focused on peace and living according to G-d's will.

At the end of our lunch, I took my box lunch trash and discarded it in a nearby trash can. I noticed my new Muslim friend couldn't be bothered by that and left the rest of his lunch as litter on the park bench. That was my first impression of what he had done. Then I remembered how important charity is in Islam. I asked Samir why he left his lunch on the park bench. He said that he couldn't eat the sandwich (because it contained a pork product), and he wasn't hungry enough to eat the apple. "It is proper to leave this good food for a less fortunate, perhaps homeless person to eat," he said.

The Islamic faith isn't an abstract thing to Samir Hantirah. Islam's focus on being charitable is a part of his everyday life. I have a lot of respect for that.

Much as dermatologists were wrong when they thought patients were regularly using their medication, my initial impression that the Muslim dermatologist was unthinkingly littering was completely misguided. We don't know or see what goes on in people's heads, so we ought to be careful when we ascribe motivations to their actions. Moreover, we can't always trust what we see. When Muslim people go to the mosque to pray for peace, we don't read about it in our news. It's not news when Palestinians go about their day-to-day routine (whatever that is) in their refugee camps. It is news, however, when any one of the billion Muslims commits some terrorist act, just as it is news in Winston-Salem if just one of Lee Garrity's 2,500 employees doesn't do his or her job right. Even if only one in a million Muslims is a terrorist, that one is the one we'll read about in our paper. It may be that associating Islam with violence is even more misguided than associating U.S. Postal Service employees with murderous work rage.

PART 3

The Insidious Effect
of Context on Perception

Visual Illusions

There are some things we just don't see, and therefore we can't say much about them with great certainty. There are many other things we do see, but they may not be representative of the full reality; basing our judgments on those observations may lead us to absurd conclusions. But even when we observe a representative sample of something, compartments can affect our perceptions of the event. To understand this, we first have to understand something about how our brains function. Visual illusions provide a fascinating window on how our brains process information. A critical feature of many illusions is that our perceptions are colored by context.

Consider one of the "simplest" illusions, the perceptions of color presented on different backgrounds. I've put the word "simplest" in quotes because our visual functioning is a very powerful and complex function of our minds. Scientists continue to explore how our brain is able to make sense of the things we see.

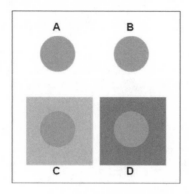

Figure 1

In the figure, two identical gray disks (A and B) are shown. One disk is inside a light square (C), and the other is inside a dark square (D). The disk inside the light square looks darker than the disk inside the dark square. This phenomenon tells us much about how we process visual information. There is an objective reality: two identical gray disks. The two gray disks send similar photons that hit the retinas of our eyes. But because one disk is presented in the context of a dark surrounding, it appears lighter in color than an identical disk that is presented in the context of a light surrounding.

The illusion is a function of how our visual system works. The retina at the back of our eyes captures photons and turns them into electrical signals that are sent to the brain. Lower portions of the brain begin to integrate these signals, sending them to higher portions of the brain to interpret them. The ultimate interpretation of the shade of the disk depends in part on the number of photons from the disk that hit the retina. The interpretation of shading also depends on other signals, including the signals that come from photons hitting other portions of the retina.

Even simple visual illusions can be fascinating. The way our perceptions can be fooled is somewhat striking. *Scientific American* has a wonderful article by Dr. Alan Gilchrist describing the complex way we perceive shades of color (Gilchrist A 2006).

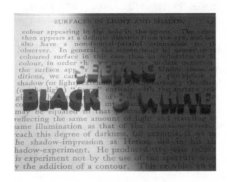

BLACK   WHITE

Figure 2a   Figure 2b

Gilchrist, author of the book *Seeing Black and White*, probes the way the mind perceives grayscale colors through the use of visual illusions. One of his most striking illusions is presented in figure 2. In figure 2A, we see black letters and white letters. The letters in the word "black" look black, and the letters in the word "white" look white. But when the context is removed in figure 2b, we can see that the white letters are actually a darker shade of gray than the black letters are!

One of the most intriguing things about these illusions is that we consciously can understand them. We can be shown that the letters in the word "white" are actually darker than the letters in the word "black." We can *know* the letters in the word "white" are darker than the letters in the word "black," but we still perceive that the letters in the word "black" are black and look darker than the letters in the word "white" in this illusion. Our perceptions happen in that amazing computer we call our brain, and we can't fully control those perceptions. We can look and look and look, knowing the white letters are darker, and still it seems that the white letters are white, and the black letters are black when we look at the picture. The context controls our perception.

There are objective realities here. We could use a computer program to measure the actual colors on the paper. We can measure the intensity of light reaching our eyes. Yet what we see in our mind's eye is a construct, a construct that the brain creates based on the objective reality that hits the retina. Much of the time, the construct provides a very good representation of reality. When it doesn't, when we see a visual illusion, it can be fun, cool, and interesting. Much like comedy, the unpredictability of illusions is entertaining.

Visual illusions are used by scientists to better understand how our brains process information. The neurons in our brain that react to visual stimuli do so in a coordinated manner that depends in part on the activity of other neurons. There is a neuron in the brain that "looks" at the color of the gray square; the color that neuron "sees" depends on how much light or dark the neurons around it are seeing. Visual perception is based on the complex workings of a network of neurons. What we see (that is to say, what we perceive) *depends on the context* in which we see it.

The Insidious Effect of Context on Our Observations

If you were to look at an atlas of the human vascular system, you'll see the heart, arteries, and veins. The arteries carry blood away from the heart, carrying needed oxygen to our tissues. Veins return the blood to the right side of the heart, which then sends the blood to the lungs to pick up oxygen again. In diagrams of the vascular system, the arteries and veins are easily distinguished: the arteries are colored red, and the veins are colored blue. This color scheme is pretty much universal.

Are veins blue in real life? It seems like they are. If you take a biology class in high school or college, you may have the opportunity to dissect an animal. When you do, you may find that the arteries are red and the veins are blue. The reason for this, however, is that to better see the blood vessels in the dissection, the vessels are injected with colored latex. According to the same convention used in the atlas diagrams, red latex is used for the arteries and blue latex for the veins.

If you look at the palm side of your wrist, you can see the veins. They too are blue. I've wondered why they are blue. I was taught that the oxygenated blood in the arteries is red, and that the deoxygenated blood in the veins is blue. While it is true that the oxygenated blood in the arteries is a bright red color, the blood in the veins is also a red color, not blue. Donate blood at the Red Cross some time. When you do, you'll see red blood come out of the vein, not anything blue. Well, if the color of the blood is red and not blue, why do the veins look blue? It's not the vein itself that is blue. If you dissect a vein without first infiltrating it with blue latex, you will see that the walls of the veins aren't blue at all. What causes the blue color we see?

Although the veins may look blue, it turns out that the veins aren't actually blue. Here's a simple experiment you can do with a digital camera and a computer (Feldman 2007). Take a picture of the vein on the palm side of your wrist, and then use photo software to assess the color of the vein. You can see an example of this experiment on the back cover of this book. Have the computer draw a line of that color on a neutral gray background. The color of the line (A) isn't blue! The computer will show it is pink. Look again at the vein on your wrist. Your eyes (actually your brain) will say the color is blue.

Next, use the software to identify the color of the skin on either side of the vein (B). The computer will again show a shade of pink. Create a square of that color and use it to replace the neutral gray background. In the context of the new background, you will see the appearance of the vein-colored line change to a shade of blue!

But if you look at your wrist, the vein still appears blue. An even simpler test can confirm that though your eyes and brain perceive blue, the vein is actually a pinkish flesh color. All this second test requires is two pieces of standard gray duct tape. Place one piece of the duct tape on each side of the vein, covering the adjacent skin. Once you see the vein all by itself, you can see its real color, a shade of pink.

Our brains are wired to recognize the world through contrasts, contrasts between an observation and its context. Orange juice may taste sweet, but a moment later—after a bowl of Cap'n Crunch cereal—it will taste tart. A cola may taste sweet, but after taking a bite of ice cream, it may taste closer to bitter. Our taste sensation is based on context.

Our brain's sense of smell is also based on contrast. When we walk into a house where someone is baking cookies or cooking with garlic, the smell can be very striking. After a while, we get used to it and don't notice it anymore. The smell is still in the air, but our brains tune it out.

Our attention to sound is also dependent on contrasts. Have you ever been in a room with an air conditioner running and not noticed it until the air conditioner stopped? The white-noise drone gets ignored. As soon as there is a change, we notice it. Normally, we might not notice silence. But when we face silence in the context of having heard noise, we easily pick it out.

This isn't to say seeing in contrast or having senses affected by context is bad. On the contrary, undoubtedly it kept our ancestors alive. Nature selected us for being able to efficiently detect the lion hiding in the grass. This feature let our primate ancestors and their ancestors reproduce. The way our brains are wired, we are exquisitely able to detect differences. My wife once detected the slightest variation between the slopes of two bookshelves that I had hung, just millimeters over several feet, from across the room. Had there been only one shelf, I would have been free and clear. Because there were two, I was in trouble. It was much easier for her to see the contrast between the two than to notice a single shelf was just slightly off level.

Even our most abstract thoughts are seen through context. We're able to motivate people to do things by giving them even a most meager reward; as long as it is a change, they notice. In the winter, a 50-degree day might feel warm; in the summer, it would be felt or experienced as unseasonably cold. We have set points for temperature, and we experience hot and cold in contrast to the set points. Our perceptions of time are dramatically affected by context. Certainly, you've experienced that time flies when you are having fun, yet it doesn't seem to move at all when you're waiting for a pot of water to boil. You may have noticed in elementary school that class seemed to take forever while watching the clock, yet recess passed in no time at all while having fun.

Our assessments of trash and treasure are affected by context. Our city provides an annual bulk item trash pickup service. One week each year we get to put out our biggest and heaviest trash items. Before the city picks up the trash, roving pickup trucks troll the neighborhood seeking what to them are treasures. One man's trash is another man's treasure because of the context in which they view the item. The entire capitalist system of buy and sell is based on the fact that different people have different perceptions of the value of things. Every sense wired into our brains, even our senses of right and wrong, are affected by the context in which we experience them.

There is an entire art devoted to the manipulation of perception. It is called magic. Great magicians are actually applied neuropsychologists. The great magicians understand how the brain perceives things, and they know how to manipulate context so that the brain perceives an illusion. The great part of magic is not so much in the trick as in the context in which that trick is presented.

The brain perceives subjectively; however, this does not mean that reality is relative. There is an objective reality out in the external world. But our internal mental perceptions of reality are all relative. If a dermatologist, the definitive expert on objective assessment of the skin, can look at a pink vein and think it is blue, you'll know that human perception, though not necessarily flawed, is certainly affected by context.

—

Abstract Perceptions Are Colored by Context

The way context affects our abstract perceptions is illustrated by the way people think in Winston-Salem, North Carolina, a small city in the southern United States. Life is good here. For an academic dermatologist, Winston-Salem offers all the advantages of both a major medical center, the Wake Forest University Baptist Medical Center, and small town life. My wife and I bought a home here within walking distance to work. Later, after having children, we moved way out to the American dream, suburbs where the homes have big yards in which the children can play. The trade-off was an eight-minute commute to work.

Winston-Salem traffic presents a nice example of perception being colored by the context of experience. I grew up just inside the Washington, DC, Beltway. Traffic on the Beltway can be nasty at times. On good days, it can be harrowing. On bad days, it is like sitting in a parking lot. To me, Winston-Salem traffic, even at its worst, is like a walk in the park. On the other hand, the city traffic of Washington, DC, now makes me sweaty and causes my heart to race.

The job of a dermatologist at Wake Forest University takes me to Mount Airy, North Carolina, one day a week. Mount Airy, the birthplace of Andy Griffith, is a small town (with a population of about 10,000), which would have been of little notice, had it not become famous for being the town on which the fictional TV town of Mayberry (on the popular and long-running *Andy Griffith Show*) was based. Mount Airy is a lovely town with wonderful people. Some of the patients I've seen there require more specialized medical services offered at the university medical center in Winston-Salem. But many of these patients react in near terror when I suggest they go to the university. It is not because they are afraid of the big hospital or of high technology medical care. "Winston-Salem?" they say, "We don't like to go there. The traffic is so bad."

The traffic in Winston-Salem is the same whether you grew up in Manhattan or in Tick Bite (an even smaller North Carolina town). How one perceives that traffic, however, does depend on where you came from and what you are accustomed. Coming from a larger, more populous city, Winston-Salem traffic seems pleasant. For some people living in more rural communities, Winston-Salem traffic might seem harrowing. The context in which a person perceives the objective reality of the number of cars on the road determines that person's perception of the traffic. Winston-Salem traffic isn't the only example Winston-Salem offers of how context affects perception.

Winston-Salem is known for its two major products, Winston and Salem cigarettes. The town's formerly prominent nickname, the Camel City, was based on its third major product, Camel cigarettes. The cigarette business, R. J. Reynolds Tobacco Company, is not what it used to be. When my wife and I moved to Winston, the influence of tobacco was completely pervasive there. Our first dermatology faculty dinner was held at a small French restaurant on the grounds of the former Reynolds estate. As we left the restaurant at the end of the meal, we noticed that where we might have expected to see a bowl of mints by the door, there was instead a bowl of loose cigarettes.

Reynolds employees served in the city and county governments. When the local school system needed judges for school science fair competitions, they called Reynolds, and Reynolds' scientists would come and volunteer. People smoked in the grocery stores. Most everyone in town worked for the tobacco company, had a family member that did, or served in a business that catered to tobacco workers. The influence of tobacco here is no longer what it used to be—our medical center is now the largest employer in town—but Winston-Salem is still more tobacco-friendly than most places. I suspect our medical center was probably among the very last medical centers in the country to become a smoke-free facility.

While the tobacco culture hasn't been entirely lost, Winston-Salem used to exhibit a strong sense of pride in tobacco. There was pride in the self-sufficient family farmer growing tobacco and in the cigarette factory worker. This was quite surprising to those of us in the health care industry. Winston-Salem was making a product that slowly killed people, but the population took pride in making a legal product and making it well. It took pride in American freedom, including the freedom to be a smoker. Winston-Salem took pride in helping those smokers in their freedom to smoke. Reynolds Tobacco had a motto: Pride in Tobacco. You could see it frequently on bumper stickers and license plates.

If there ever was a case of context affecting perception, here it is. Cigarette smoke is a carcinogen. Cigarettes cause emphysema, cancer, and cardiovascular disease. Cigarettes are an addictive product that lead to strokes in some people and amputations in others. Many people would see cigarettes as evil. People in Winston-Salem took pride in tobacco.

The human brain is an amazing organ. In some visual illusions, we can look at static lines on a sheet of paper, and it seems as though they are moving even though we know they can't possibly be moving. We can look at a pinkish-colored vein on our wrist and see blue. And we can look at a product that damages people's health and take pride in making it. All our perceptions are colored by context. This is how our brains are wired. Perception is not something we easily control. People in Winston-Salem knew the objective information about the health effects of tobacco just like everyone else, yet they still had completely different perceptions about the manufacture, sale, and use of tobacco products. This isn't just true of people in Winston-Salem. Some people in Michigan probably have similar feelings about auto emission standards while some people in Las Vegas might have similar feelings about the gambling industry. The taxes one perceives as "fair" might well depend on one's wealth or the sources of one's income.

Whatever we look at, we need to consider how our context affects our perceptions. Many times the differences of opinion that people hold come simply from seeing the same objective reality and mentally interpreting it in very different ways.

Patients' Impressions
of Their Doctors

The way patients perceive their doctors is affected by context. I had been practicing for a few years before our medical center began doing regular patient satisfaction surveys in the dermatology clinic. The surveys were enlightening to me. I didn't know what patients thought of me or the care they received from me. I thought most of them were pretty happy though. The surveys showed that most of my patients actually loved the care I was giving them. A few, however, thought I was terrible. The only way to find out what patients thought was to ask them. To achieve the goal of making sure all patients thought they received great medical care, I needed feedback.

I started using the *www.DrScore.com* online patient-satisfaction survey Web site to get regular feedback from patients. At the end of an office visit, I would ask patients to go online and give me feedback on what they liked and what they didn't like about their visit. About nineteen out of every twenty patients said I was doing a very good job. The praise was a great boost to my ego. But then one in every twenty or so patients said I was terrible. The comments that hurt the most were the ones that said I was uncaring.

Like other doctors, I spent years at hard work in college allowing me to get into medical school. I worked very hard in medical school not just to graduate but to make sure I would give patients great care. I spent three more years specializing in dermatology and have continued my education ever since. When patients said on their surveys that I didn't care about them, at first I was angry. I had devoted so much of my life to medicine because, like other doctors, I cared deeply about my patients and their well-being.

Then I realized that it wasn't patients' fault that I didn't appear caring to them. They can't see how I feel internally, so they base their sense of my caring attitude on the things they do see. When it comes to skin problems, I can make accurate diagnosis very, very quickly. Many rashes are like the Mona Lisa or a helicopter—after you've seen them, you recognize them again immediately. With all my training, I know exactly how to treat these rashes. For some patients, I can make the diagnosis and prescribe the right treatment in seconds. I might hand these patients a prescription and leave the room feeling very proud of myself for knowing exactly what the patient had, for having given them the best possible treatment, and for having given them great medical care. Unfortunately, when I am that efficient, I may leave the patient thinking that I didn't take time to do a thorough examination, that I didn't take time to get a full history, and that consequently I didn't care about the patient.

Sometimes, the context the patient brings to the visit may affect their view of me. If you come to our dermatology clinic, the first thing you see is our waiting room. There are glass windows and blinds behind which the office reception staff sits. This gives the reception area a look like the reception desk at a local jail or some other uncaring business that at any moment might shut itself off from you in a most uncaring way. There are several signs up about our financial policies—our copayment policy, our return check policy, our insurance card policy, and our credit card policy. While our intent in posting these signs may have been to help patients, the signs may leave some patients with the impression that I care more about payments than I do about helping patients get well.[4] And if patients come on a day when I've fallen behind, the long wait to be seen compounds the problem, reinforcing patients' sense that I just don't care about them.

My father, Ed Feldman, needed a new doctor. His internist had retired. In his search for a new doctor, often the first question he was asked was, "What kind of insurance do you have?" When that was the first question he heard, he felt as though that practice must care more about money than about patients. What he wanted to hear was, "We would love to help you. What kind of medical problem do you have?" I'm sure all the medical practices my father contacted care deeply about their patients. Unfortunately, they may not be letting all their patients know they care.

The context that patients have affects how they perceive their doctors. Patients don't have a direct view of all the years doctors spend in training nor of the continuing education efforts physicians go to in order to make sure they are giving patients the best possible medical care. It would be a shame if doctors set a context that leaves patients thinking doctors care more about dollars than about our patients' well-being.

I'm a very happy dermatologist. I have a smile on my face when I see people. Most of my patients tell me they like that, that they like the friendly, caring attention I give them. Some of my patients see that smile and think I'm laughing at them. Despite many years of effort studying to be a good doctor and making sure my patients

---

4. We ought to have a sign that says, "We appreciate the trust you put in us and work to give you the best medical care."

get the best possible care, some patients perceive me as uncaring. Whether they see me as caring or uncaring may depend as much on context (their previous experiences as well as the staff and facilities of my office) as it does with my own behavior.

Magicians understand that what their audience perceives depends on the context in which the magician presents his or her illusions. In describing the craft of magic, Henning Nelms (1969) wrote,

> As the object of the effect is to convince the spectators, their interpretation of the evidence is the only thing that counts. When the effect consists in taking a cannon ball from an empty hat, the audience must believe that the hat is empty and that the cannon ball is heavy. If the spectators accept this, a one-ounce half-globe of papier-mâché is as good as a twenty-pound iron sphere; if they regard the ball as an imitation, iron is no better than papier-mâché.

What the audience sees is a black round object. Whether they think it is a cannonball made of iron or a cheap piece of papier-mâché depends on the context in which they see it.

Dermatologists are nearly always able to give patients the right diagnosis and the right treatment for their skin diseases. Patients have a hard time knowing whether diagnoses and treatments are correct or not. Whether patients perceive that their medical care is great medical care or not is a lot like how they perceive the iron ball or a papier-mâché ball in the magic trick. If the context of the office visit suggests lousy care, patient may perceive lousy care even when the care is good.

Whatever business a person is in, he or she must be attentive to the context the business presents to customers. To be a most effective physician, doctors need to understand how patients' perceptions are affected by context. Even in a relationship as intimate as the patient-physician relationship, there may be considerable misunderstanding. These misunderstandings are magnified when people are separated into different groups, as they are when people in the different compartments of the health care system perceive each other.

Impressions of the Health Care System

The health care system in the United States is huge and complex. Within the health care system, there are many different compartments. The context held by people in different compartments causes plenty of conflict. Consider the people in the following health care compartments, each of which includes many subcategories of personnel. First, we have doctors; doctors are caring professionals devoted to helping people. Second, there's the pharmaceutical and medical supply industry; this industry is composed of companies that devote huge resources and take great risks to develop and market treatments that doctors use to make people's lives better. And third, there's the health insurance industry; this industry consists of organizations that pay for the health care that patients use.

Each of the major components of the health care system are made up of people, people who have chosen a career in industries that help ill people get well. Yet people working in any one of these compartments might question the motivations of the people in another. While health insurance companies are in the business of helping people pay for health care, the vehemence with which doctors, politicians, and other people deride health insurers is staggering.

Consider Amy Hamaker. Amy works in the durable medical equipment industry, at a company that specializes in complex custom wheelchairs. As Amy puts it, "The retail cost of some of these would make your head spin. I submit the claims for this equipment. Just today I had to have a colleague adjust a bill from a $36,000 custom power wheelchair" (Hamaker 2008). Amy deals directly with health insurance companies. It is frustrating work at times. "The majority of the smaller claims are paid within a reasonable time frame. The bigger ones can take up to two years to be fully paid at the allowed amount. I have heard every excuse in the book for lack of payment. I've seen what my employer also pays out for the other durable medical equipment we carry (beds, oxygen, etc) and along with everything else he has to dish out, I can understand why our management team pushes us to get our claims paid. Reimbursement rates keep going down. In the durable medical equipment industry, when this happens, quality products become less available."

Amy is a wonderful person who devotes her work life to helping quadriplegic patients get medical equipment that helps them function. Her view of health insurers is pretty bleak. She thinks insurance companies appear "greedy, making so much profit from people when they are at the most vulnerable time of their lives. Their objective is to control the flow of money accrued from insurance premiums (almost like a glorified bank). Insurance companies have clinicians on their staff that are actually rewarded bonuses (sometimes hefty ones) when they save the insurance companies money by denying a claim," she says. One particular example stands out in her mind, that of an insurance company physician executive who denied a claim resulting in a patient's death. Amy says the denial resulted in the physician getting a pay raise and promotion. She sees that health insurers' goals are to make money, not to help patients. Amy questions why health insurance company executives make so much money when that money could be used to take care of patients. Amy wonders how health insurers can live with themselves considering how their only goal is to make money at the expense of sick people.

But let's consider the possibility that at the health insurance company there is another Amy. The Amy working for the health insurer says, "I get the claims from the doctors and pharmaceutical companies. What they charge us would make your head spin! We're doing our best to control costs so that people can afford health insurance. But they charge $36,000 for a wheelchair! Drug companies try to charge us over $100,000/year for some of the new drugs, and that's for a single patient! The doctors and the CEOs of the drug companies are raking in the money, and the money is coming from patients. We insurers don't print money. We just help distribute it from a pool of people who need care to the pool of doctors and drug companies that only care about the almighty dollar and not about the patient. How do the doctors and drug companies and durable medical equipment manufacturers sleep at night!"

The views of doctors, insurers, and drug companies are probably symmetric and could be described in rather similar terms. Each sees the other two as the problem; each group sees itself in a positive light. I'm a doctor and know my perspective pretty well. Doctors care deeply about their patients' health and don't have trouble sleeping at night, even though we tend to get paid well for what we do. In contrast, doctors often have dim views of drug companies and health insurers. Issues like the Vioxx controversy (Kweder 2004) and the ever-rising cost of medications may stand out when thinking about drug companies, even though on a day-to-day basis, drug companies give doctors the tools we use to improve patients' health and well-being. When health insurers pay the bills—which they tend to do day in and day out—we don't pay it much attention, much like the steady drone of an air conditioner. The few times when insurers deny coverage for some requested treatment stand out in our minds as does the steady drone of an air conditioner that suddenly cuts off.

I bet the people who work at drug companies think they are doing humanity a great service by searching for and making available the drugs that make people's lives better. At the pharmaceutical companies that make the new, life-altering treatments for psoriasis, I've met people who see themselves as patient advocates, as partners in helping doctors improve patients' lives. I bet the people at the insurance company sleep very well too, thinking that they are doing humanity a great service by helping people pay a fair price for quality health care. The pharmaceutical benefit managers I've met expressed a deep commitment to helping patients get the care they need. Yet when people in any of these "compartments" look at the folks in the other compartment, they think those other folks are "bastards who are only in it for the money."

I had an experience that drove this point home. I met with a group of pharmacy benefit managers to educate them about psoriasis treatment. Pharmacy benefit managers help control what drugs are on or off an insurer's formulary. They are in a great position to help doctors make sure psoriasis patients get the care they need. They are also in a great position to really foul things up if they don't understand psoriasis, its impact on people, the great diversity of treatment options, and how these treatments are used. Many doctors believe that health insurance companies don't really care much about patients, even less about psoriasis, except as far as it helps them make money.

On the contrary, the pharmacy benefit managers at this meeting, representing a broad range of private insurance companies across the country, were extremely interested in psoriasis treatment. They didn't seem to want to prevent all patients from getting expensive treatment. They did ask for information and guidance to help make sure that patients were treated appropriately and that the criteria insurers had in place for using the new expensive medicines were sensible. Seeing these managers' interest in coming up with policies that really did help people was heartening. As far as these particular managers go, it seemed to me that doctors' dim view of them was misplaced.

At the break, one of the attendees approached me. He was concerned that drug companies were heavily marketing new expensive treatments to dermatologists. "Drug companies are bringing lunches to dermatologists every day," he said. "And dermatologists aren't going to want the lunches to end." He thought free lunches were driving dermatologists to prescribe drugs that cost $20,000 per year per patient. He fervently believed that there were daily free lunches that were encouraging dermatologists to fight efforts to control use of these expensive drugs.

I gently suggested to him that in reality dermatologists' motivation is their interest in helping their patients have access to the drugs they need. At the same time, I was thinking about how the idea this pharmacy benefit manager had was *completely and utterly ridiculous.* I have no idea why he thinks that dermatologists are getting catered lunches every day. I'm not, and none of the dermatologists I know are. To whatever extent salespeople may be bringing lunch to doctors' offices, those lunches are not going to make a doctor prescribe a $20,000-a-year drug to someone who doesn't need it. It is almost completely incomprehensible that someone would think that doctors would want to see open access to expensive drugs on insurers' formularies primarily because they like getting lunch brought to the office. The only way this is comprehensible is by understanding how warped people's perceptions can be of people in other compartments.

The effect of compartments is amazing. A thoroughly intelligent, well balanced, high-functioning medical professional, a doctor of pharmacy, can end up with completely false ideas about doctors. This pharmacy benefit manager's warped impression of dermatologists seems to mirror the warped perceptions doctors have of people working in the health insurance industry. People in one compartment have a tendency to think ill of those in another. Sometimes the ideas people have of people in another compartment are completely and utterly ridiculous.

Our health care system is not perfect. It is certainly costly, and some people don't have good access to care. At the same time, the health care system has a lot going for it, not the least of which are many caring people—doctors, nurses, administrators (yes, even administrators), insurers, and drug manufacturers—who work hard so that patients get great medical care.

Patient Safety

Patient safety is a critical issue to all physicians, but often, physicians in one specialty don't recognize the commitment to patient safety of colleagues in another. Misperceptions may be caused by the experiences, selection bias, and context in which physicians interpret their observations. On May 13, 1999, the *New England Journal of Medicine* published a story about five people whose deaths from liposuction procedures between 1993 and 1998 were reported to the Office of Chief Medical Examiner of the City of New York (Rao 1999). The authors of the study thought several of the deaths were caused by complications related to anesthesia. National Public Radio covered the story immediately (National Public Radio 1999). Dr. Lucien Leape, a surgeon and Harvard School of Public Health policy analyst, was asked to comment on the findings. When cosmetic surgery is performed in a doctor's office instead of a hospital, anesthesia is often given by the cosmetic surgeon and not by a specially trained anesthesiologist. "When it's done this way, the risk appears to be much higher than most of us ever thought. It raises a serious question about whether anesthetics should be given in the office situation," he said.

The safety of office surgery was questioned in greater detail by an investigative team in the Department of Anesthesiology and the

H. Lee Moffitt Cancer Center and Research Institute in Tampa, Florida (Vila 2003). The team had the benefit of using a very large database of adverse events associated with surgical procedures done in doctors' offices in Florida. Florida has been a leading state in requiring reporting of adverse events and registration of offices in which advanced surgeries are done. After highly publicized office surgery deaths in Florida, the Florida Board of Medicine placed a moratorium on doing advanced surgery in the office and implemented an adverse event monitoring system. After the moratorium was lifted, the adverse event reporting system continued to collect data on deaths and other adverse events associated with office surgeries.

The Florida anesthesiology team reviewed adverse incidents reported to the Florida Board of Medicine for surgical procedures in physicians' offices between April 1, 2000, and April 1, 2002. They compared the results to the rate of reported adverse events that occurred in accredited surgical centers in Florida in the year 2000. They found that the risk of adverse incidents and death was about *ten times higher* in the office setting compared to the accredited surgical centers.

Anesthesiologists were dumbfounded that other physicians would permit office surgery to be done without appropriate safeguards. Writing in the *Anesthesia Patient Safety Foundation Newsletter*, Dr. Robert Morell described how profit was responsible for the growth in office-based anesthesia, and Dr. Ervin Moss reported that patient safety and the saving of lives didn't seem to impress self-serving doctors who saw regulations as a threat to their financial bottom line (Morell 2000; Moss 2000). Dr. Rudolph de Jong, a leading expert on local anesthesia, described the startling mortality associated with liposuction and concluded that anesthesiologists should be consulted or engaged for patient safety monitoring during major liposuction or conscious sedation procedures, wherever those procedures are done.

Plastic surgeons too were engaged in the debate. They saw that dermatologists and other specialists could do cosmetic surgery in their offices without even having hospital privileges for doing those surgeries. Using patient safety as justification, surgeons promoted regulations that would require physicians to have hospital privileges for a procedure before a physician would be allowed to perform that surgery in their offices.

To dermatologists, it wasn't hard to see that it was the anesthesiologists and surgeons who were being self-serving. A closer look at the *New England Journal of Medicine* article revealed that all five reported deaths were associated with procedures done by surgeons (plastic surgeons in four of the five cases), not by dermatologists. Anesthesiologists were actually present at the surgery for all five of these patients. Using the *New England Journal of Medicine* data to promote having an anesthesiologist present seemed a bit of a stretch to the dermatology community.

A closer look at the analysis of Florida adverse event data was equally enlightening. The investigators knew how many deaths and adverse events happened in doctor's offices from the adverse event database, but that database didn't tell how many procedures were done. The anesthesiology team estimated the number of procedures from those reported by offices "registered" to do *complicated* surgical procedures. But registered offices accounted for only a small percentage of offices doing surgery as most procedures were minor. To get the rates of deaths and adverse events, the investigators included deaths and other adverse events from *all* offices but used as a denominator only the number of procedures done in *registered* offices. I was among a team of dermatologists who recognized the error in the analysis, reanalyzed the data, and found that death and adverse event rates were actually considerably *lower* in doctors' offices than they were in the accredited surgical centers (Venkat 2004).

As primarily an office-based specialty, dermatologists often have no need for hospital privileges. Dermatologists could see how plastic surgeons and anesthesiologists were trying to use the flawed analysis of Florida adverse event reports to support proposed hospital privileges regulations, regulations whose effect would be to block dermatologists from doing cosmetic surgery. Hospital privileges were given out by panels of hospital-based surgeons who would be able to block other specialties from doing office-based surgery. Keeping the surgery in the hospitals would also mean more fees for anesthesiologists.

The regulations being promoted by surgeons rankled dermatologists, and no one was more rankled than Dr. Brett Coldiron. Coldiron is a dermatologist specializing in skin surgery. He provides that care out of his own office. Coldiron is an imposing, larger-than-life figure, easily capable of commanding attention. He knew dermatologic surgeons are among the brightest and most hardworking physicians and are devoted to their patients. Most dermatologists, although upset and angry about the proposed regulations, took no action. Coldiron initiated an effort to look more closely at the Florida data to assess the surgeons' arguments that doctors be required to have hospital privileges to perform surgical procedures in their offices.

Coldiron and his team contacted each doctor who reported a death or adverse event to get the details about their board certification and hospital privileges status. In December of 2007, his group reported their findings based on seven years of the Florida data (Coldiron 2007). They found 31 deaths and 143 procedure-related complications. Plastic surgeons were responsible for 83 percent of the cosmetic surgery deaths and complications. Coldiron concluded that requiring physician board certification or physician hospital privileges would not likely increase safety because most physicians already had these credentials, and physicians without these credentials were not responsible for a disproportionate share of the deaths or adverse events.

From the dermatologists' perspective, it appeared that all the anesthesiologists and surgeons cared about was their own wallets and not about patient safety. Dermatologists knew that they had patients' best interest at heart and knew that the procedures done by dermatologists were safe and effective. The attacks on dermatology had to be motivated by something else. It seemed clear the anesthesiologists didn't want to be cut out of providing anesthesia services, which could happen as more and more surgery was being done in doctors' offices instead of hospitals. Dermatologists also saw how surgeons wanted regulations that would prevent office-based physicians, including dermatologists, from doing lucrative cosmetic surgery cases.

I had a chance to talk directly with surgeons and anesthesiologists about the office-based surgery issue. I could not have been more wrong about them. They were deeply passionate in their commitment to patient safety. It was clear that a turf battle about who did surgery was not their primary concern at all. The anesthesiologists exuded a deep pride in their successful efforts to reduce injuries and deaths associated with general anesthesia. They were unfamiliar with what dermatologists did in their offices. The anesthesiologists never saw any of the patients dermatologists successfully managed without the help of an anesthesiologist, yet they did see the very few who experienced a problem that required the intervention of an anesthesiologist. As we saw with dermatologists and family physicians, the anesthesiologists' experience with patients who had surgery done by a dermatologist was that there was always an untoward outcome; anesthesiologists never saw the dermatologists' many successes. Anesthesiologists wanted patients to be safe, and their perception was that dermatologists were engaged in unsafe practices and cared more about money than patients.

—

In my dermatology compartment, I had thought very poorly of the anesthesia team that had studied the risk of office-based surgery. They had claimed there was a tenfold higher risk of adverse events and deaths for surgeries done in doctors' offices as compared to surgeries done in surgical centers. That made no sense to me or other dermatologists. In dermatology, we rarely if ever see such adverse events. Surely the anesthesiology research team must have recognized the error and knew they had been presenting inaccurate information, I thought. Yet after speaking with anesthesiologists directly, it was clear the tenfold error they had made in calculating the safety rates of office procedures wasn't done maliciously; the findings probably fit with their experiences. They never saw any of our successes, only the rare problems.

There were plastic surgeons who looked at the *New England Journal of Medicine* report and thought patients ought to see a board-certified plastic surgeon for liposuction and not some lesser specialty. These surgeons probably perceived that they did liposuction safely but didn't trust the training of other specialists. Their thoughts were colored by their experience of seeing only the failures of other specialties, not their successes. Other surgeons I talked to also seemed to have no interest in the office-based practices of dermatologists whatsoever. These surgeons expressed heartfelt concerns about patient welfare and described how surgeons regulate each other. If a surgeon is found to be operating while intoxicated or otherwise impaired, their hospital privileges are revoked. The surgeons I spoke with wanted to see regulations requiring hospital privileges before a physician could perform surgery in the office in order to prevent an impaired surgeon whose hospital privileges had been revoked from going across the street to his or her office and doing surgery there.

Dermatologists, surgeons, and anesthesiologists had ill-conceived attitudes about the others. The symmetry in their views was uncanny. None of the three seemed to recognize the deep, abiding commitment to patients that the others had. None could see past their own compartment, much less into the heads of their colleagues. Their experiences were colored by the adverse outcomes they had observed and the fact that they never saw each others' successes. Within their compartments, they talked among themselves with a growing distrust of the other groups. The lack of interdisciplinary communication prevented them from recognizing their common commitment to patients' health and well-being. Had they just sat down and talked with one another, many of the misconceptions probably could have been averted.

While it isn't easy, efforts to enhance patient safety at the level of state medical societies will require physicians of different specialties to collaborate, putting aside our biases and preconceived notions. Making ill-informed statements about how some specialties care more about profit than patients is not only wrong; it also engenders needless animosity that makes collaboration more difficult.

Five liposuction deaths reported in a medical journal tell us very little; we don't know how many deaths may have gone unreported, and we don't know how many cases without death or injury were done. Do the reported deaths represent the tip of an iceberg of unreported events, or were they one-in-a-million unforeseeable and unpreventable outcomes? We can't tell. All medical specialties should be able to agree that mandatory reporting of surgical deaths and other adverse events is an essential step in promoting the shared goal of all these specialty groups: safe and effective patient care.

It is amazing how quickly compartments change our views of the world. All these doctors went to medical school together. But sometime after starting their residency, they affiliate with a particular specialty. The doctors in dermatology, anesthesiology, and surgery all knew themselves to be committed to giving patients the best possible care, but they had a very hard time seeing that this was true of colleagues in other specialties. Each thought themselves to be almost saintly and thought that the others were basically greedy and uncaring.

Perhaps we've been conditioned from youth to see conflicts in black-and-white terms of *good* and *evil*. The themes of so many Disney movies and cartoons are based on that theme. In the real world, however, conflict often involves misconceptions between those who see themselves as *good* on one side and those that see themselves as *good* on the other side. Even in the most hideous divorce battles, probably each side sees the other side in the wrong and themselves in the right (yet presumably at some point in the past, both saw something positive in the other).

For the doctors, getting past seeing each other as evil and working together to promote great medical care is probably a lot easier than many of the other compartment-caused conflicts we see today.

"Evil" Tanning-Bed Operators

Dermatologists' perceptions of tanning-bed operators gives us a good opportunity to consider how context affects people's perceptions of others as *evil*. Dermatologists see a lot of patients with skin cancer. Some skin cancers are caught early and are easily removed, leaving only a small scar. Other skin cancers are larger, and the treatment required to cure them results in substantial scarring and damage. A bad skin cancer can eat off a nose or an ear, or worse. The worst skin cancers, melanomas, can kill a person. Dermatologists have seen many bad outcomes from skin cancer. One of the things about skin cancer that most frustrates dermatologists is that skin cancer should be preventable. Tanning-bed operators are, from a dermatologist's perspective, part of the problem.

Skin cancers are caused by exposure to ultraviolet radiation. Outdoor work and recreational activities expose people to ultraviolet light from the sun. These rays damage the skin. They damage the genetic material, the DNA, in skin cells causing skin cancers to develop. Light skin color lets more of the damaging rays through, so people with fairer complexions are at greater risk from ultraviolet light. Dermatologists would like to see patients wear hats and advise patients to use sunscreen to help reduce the risk of skin cancer. Dermatologists' job isn't just treating skin cancers; dermatologists also want to prevent skin cancers from developing in the first place.

Dermatologists would like people to be more careful in how they let themselves be exposed to ultraviolet light. Dermatologists actively campaign for safe sun exposure behavior, encourage people to use sunscreen, wear protective clothing, and avoid being outdoors in the middle of the day. You may have seen advertisements from the American Academy of Dermatology warning patients about the risks for skin cancer and how to avoid them.

One of dermatologists' chief concerns in the fight against skin cancer is the ultraviolet light people get from indoor tanning. Indoor tanning has been one of the fastest-growing industries in the United States. To dermatologists' eyes, indoor tanning is a poorly regulated carcinogen exposing young people to an unnecessary risk of skin cancer.

Indoor tanning has no medical benefit for the typical user, at least none recognized by many dermatologists. There is a controversy about whether there are potential beneficial effects of indoor tanning on vitamin D levels. Dermatologists believe that even if there is a benefit from getting more vitamin D, people could get the benefit by taking an oral vitamin D supplement without having to injure the skin. Indoor tanning damages people's skin and puts people at greater risk of developing skin cancer. Many dermatologists think that the indoor tanning industry is a problem, that indoor tanning ought to be regulated, and that the people working in the tanning industry who would expose their customers—sometimes children—to harmful ultraviolet radiation just to make a buck are *evil*.

Dermatologists' views on the issue are often quite passionate. Having seen so many patients with skin cancers, dermatologists know that tanning is a big problem (of course, the people who use tanning beds and who don't have a problem from them don't tend to come to the dermatologist). Seeing a single patient die of melanoma is enough to make dermatologists question why society even allows indoor tanning parlors to exist. Some in dermatology have devoted considerable time and energy to better protect the public from the evils of tanning. The national organization of dermatologists, the American Academy of Dermatology, has been active in discouraging indoor tanning (American Academy of Dermatology 2008).

Indoor tanning adds needless risk to people's lives in exchange for an apparent cosmetic benefit, darker skin. Offering such a service is, to at least some dermatologists, morally repugnant. In some situations, it is so bad that dermatologists think the government should step in and do something about it. The American Academy of Dermatology Association opposes indoor tanning. The association supports an outright ban on the production and sale of indoor tanning equipment for nonmedical purposes (American Academy of Dermatology Association 2008).

At the same time that organized dermatology is working to reduce people's use of indoor tanning beds, the American Academy of Dermatology is promoting dermatologists' skills in providing cosmetic dermatology services. In the United States, there seems to be an almost unlimited demand for improving one's image. Patients' are willing to pay hundreds or thousands of dollars for cosmetic services. Many doctors (and even nonphysicians) have begun to tap into people's desire to look better. Millions of Botox procedures are done every year. Dermatologists, with their detailed understanding of the skin, promote themselves as a particularly good choice of doctor for people seeking a cosmetic procedure. Dermatologists offer a wide range of cosmetic surgery procedures, treatments, and services. Some dermatologists have opened medical spas devoted to promoting cosmetic services

—

alongside the medical dermatology services provided in the dermatologist's office.

On the one hand, dermatologists condemn the indoor tanning industry as evil while on the other hand, dermatologists are promoting themselves as the doctors to see for cosmetic surgery treatment. Is there a contradiction here? The benefit of cosmetic surgery isn't all that different than what indoor tanning-bed operators offer their customers. Some people perceive they look better with a tan. They may feel more self-confident. Society may look on tanned people more positively. These are the same claims offered by proponents of cosmetic surgery for the value they offer patients.

The benefits of cosmetic surgery and tanning aren't all that different. Neither are the risks. Indoor tanning causes an aging of the skin—wrinkles, leathery skin, ugly discolorations—and and an increased risk of skin cancer. There may be an increased risk of death from melanoma caused by tanning too. Cosmetic surgery also has risks. The procedures most dermatologists perform (such as Botox injections for wrinkles and chemical peels for other forms of photoaging) are fairly low risk but not completely risk free. Many procedures have a risk of scarring. Some cosmetic surgery procedures have more serious risks, including even death.

I'm not aware of any quantitative comparison of the risks of indoor tanning compared to the risk of cosmetic surgery. It is clear that both provide "cosmetic" benefit, and both have risks. What is notable is how different dermatologists' impressions can be of the person providing the service. Dermatologists may perceive cosmetic surgeons to be highly qualified professionals and tanning-bed operators as greedy opportunists who are willing to hurt people. The American Academy of Dermatology promotes a ban on indoor tanning, but it doesn't promote a ban on cosmetic surgery.

The effects of compartments—there are things we just don't see, there are things we do see that we can't trust, and context affects our perceptions—radically affect how dermatologists perceive tanning-bed operators and cosmetic surgeons. Dermatologists typically don't know the tanning parlor operators personally. Being in a different compartment, it may be easy to think the tanning parlor operators only care about money, even though the tanning-bed operators may feel good about providing a service people want and making their customers happy. Dermatologists also may not recognize how much benefit some people perceive from tanning; dermatologists don't perceive the benefit of looking darker even though many other people do. Moreover, dermatologists' experience tells them that tanning is horrible for you. All the problems associated with tanning get seen in the dermatologists' compartment while none of the far larger number of people without problems are noticed. The apparent risk of tanning seems high to dermatologists because every patient who comes in because of their tanning comes because tanning caused something bad to happen.

Context also affects the difference between how dermatologists perceive tanning versus how they perceive cosmetic surgery. While indoor tanning doesn't provide any direct financial benefit to the physician, performing cosmetic surgery does. In a time when insurers are paying less and less for office visits, a cash-paying patient seeking cosmetic services may be most welcome. Indeed, patients seem to be able to get into a dermatologist's office much quicker for cosmetic issues than they are if they have a medical skin problem (Resneck 2007). Context may lead a dermatologist to recognize that they are providing their patients a lot of benefit at low risk, something dermatologists don't perceive about indoor tanning.

Tanning is bad for the skin. I don't recommend people go to a tanning bed (unless perhaps they need it for some medical indication like psoriasis). I also don't push people to have some cosmetic procedure that they don't need. Both tanning operators and cosmetic surgeons are giving people something they desire, something that has risks, and something that is not medically indicated. When dermatologists cater to patients' requests for cosmetic services, it really isn't all that different from what tanning-bed operators do. Tanning-bed operators aren't evil. Tanning-bed operators may care about their customers as much as dermatologists care about their patients. Dermatologists' perceptions that tanning-bed operators are evil are caused by the effects of compartments on how people perceive the world around them.

How Different People View Their Psoriasis

We can make objective observations of some things, but our impressions may still be colored by context. Our judgments are subjective. When people look at skin disease, their subjective judgments about the rash can be very different. The diverse ways different people convert objective observations into subjective judgments can cause conflict, even when both parties are good, caring people.

Psoriasis can be a horrible condition that covers much of the body. It can be very itchy and sore. It can get on the palms of hands and soles of feet and limit people's ability to function. Fortunately, the majority of patients with psoriasis have just a few spots.

Consider for a moment the patient who has just a few small spots located on their elbows and knees. The spots may not even itch or burn. How bad is this kind of psoriasis?

If you were to define how bad the disease is by how much of the body is covered, you'd probably say this is mild psoriasis. If you define how bad the disease is by how much it affects one's ability to function, you might also say this is mild psoriasis. If you considered the other symptoms of the disease, the itching and soreness, you might say this patient has mild psoriasis. But none of these measures fully characterize how bad the psoriasis is because they don't take into account how much the psoriasis is bothering the patient.

Certainly many patients with this degree of psoriasis aren't bothered by the disease at all. On the other hand, a young adult, particularly a self-conscious one, might think the presence of the lesions would affect other people's impression of him or her. A person with even a few spots of psoriasis might be concerned that the lesions would affect his or her ability to have intimate relationships with others. Depending on their circumstances and idiosyncrasies, some people might find psoriasis to be no more than a minor nuisance while others could find it devastating.

There is a tendency among doctors to look at the lesions on a somewhat objective basis, to see how red, thick, and scaly they are and to recommend treatment accordingly. If I saw a patient with psoriasis spots on their elbows and knees, I might offer a variety of different topical medications to rub on the spots. Some patients with psoriasis on their elbows and knees, however, might feel their condition warranted much more aggressive treatment. They might feel that unless the lesions were totally and completely gone that they are still marked by the disease and the stigma it carries. They might feel that potent treatments that affect the immune system and that carry a risk of serious infection would be warranted.

I share patients' concerns about their psoriasis and their general well-being. There have been times when I've weighed the potential risks and benefits of a treatment and told the patient, "No, the risk of that treatment isn't warranted given the severity of the condition." Sometimes patients accept this; other times they think I am an uncaring jerk for not giving them a prescription for the treatment they want. I understand where they are coming from. I understand that their perception of the illness is different from mine. Within reason, I'm willing to go along with their perceptions. But because I care about them, sometimes I say no. I don't do it because I'm uncaring, but I can see why they would think otherwise. Even when there is a caring relationship between people, even when their ultimate goals are the same, misconceptions and conflict are possible. In fact, there are times when the *most caring* people are misled by the limitations of their compartments and are at the center of conflicts.

Isotretinoin: How Different People View a Potent Acne Treatment

Dermatologists are caring physicians who work hard to give their patients the best possible medical care. In dermatology, we're used to people questioning whether we are really doctors or not. A couple of Seinfeld episodes made that very clear. Yes, we do take care of skin cancer. There are other important things we do, one of which is taking care of teenagers with severe, scarring acne. Sometimes dermatologists' efforts to care for these patients bump up against the goals of other caring people.

As a teen, I had but a few, intermittent acne bumps. Each one was, for me, a crisis of gargantuan proportions. So I sometimes wonder how teenagers with very severe acne manage to get through the day. I'm talking about patients with "pizza face," people with acne so severe that it will leave them scarred—at the very least physically and possibly emotionally—for life.

Fortunately, dermatologists are very good at managing severe acne. The primary reason for that is because we have a drug, isotretinoin (commonly called by its original brand name,

Accutane, and now available in generic formulations) that can cure almost everyone with severe acne. Isotretinoin works when other drugs fail. It usually works even in the most severe cases.

Isotretinoin isn't perfect. It has some potential for serious side effects. Rarely, it can cause depression, though almost without doubt, it prevents (by curing severe acne) far, far more cases of depression than it causes. The biggest problem with isotretinoin is that it is a teratogen. A teratogen is a chemical that causes birth defects. In the case of isotretinoin, these can be profoundly severe birth defects. This isn't much of a problem when treating teenage boys because they tend not to get pregnant. Teratogenicity, however, is a *major* limitation for treating teenage girls with severe acne.

Dermatologists go to great lengths to use isotretinoin judiciously, cautiously, and responsibly. We do our best to make sure the women taking the drug don't get pregnant. Unfortunately, some women who take isotretinoin do become pregnant. Largely because of this, there have been efforts to make isotretinoin more difficult for patients to get and more difficult for physicians to prescribe. There have even been suggestions that the drug should be completely removed from the market in the United States.

The potential that isotretinoin would be removed from the market is a cause for great concern among dermatologists. We see many patients with severe, deforming, scarring acne. We desperately want to help these patients and prevent the permanent scarring. Isotretinoin is our best drug for that, an essential treatment option. Other people may see things differently. They may never have known a patient with truly horrendous acne. They may be more familiar with birth defects. Some pediatricians and members of lay organizations may have devoted their lives to preventing birth defects.

The iPledge program was instituted by the Food and Drug Administration to help track the pregnancies associated with isotretinoin exposure and to reduce such exposures (Hill 2006). At first, the program was extraordinarily cumbersome. It remains cumbersome but perhaps somewhat less so than it was at first.

Part of the initial problem with iPledge was slow phone service. Dermatologists' office staff would make calls to get patients started on the drug and might be left on hold for twenty minutes to an hour. An hour wait on the telephone is a completely objective thing. It is sixty minutes long. We can quantify it. We know exactly what it is. Let us consider for a moment how different people might view a one-hour wait on the telephone.

To the dermatologist caring for a patient with severe scarring acne, an hour wait on the phone to get the patient started on treatment appears to be an extraordinary waste of time and resources. It may seem like an insult to the skills, care, and professionalism of the dermatologist, whose right to prescribe isotretinoin is being questioned. Given the severity of the patient's condition, the hour wait on the phone seems to be a travesty, limiting the access of patients to a drug they desperately need. To the nurse making the call, it is exasperating enough to "make one feel like pulling one's hair out."

Would a member of the March of Dimes, an organization devoted to reducing birth defects, see things the same way? Of course not. They may look at this and think to themselves, "An hour wait to prevent a birth defect? Well, that doesn't sound like too much. Maybe it should be longer. If an hour wait to get isotretinoin helps prevent even one birth defect, it is well worth it."

An hour wait on the phone is a completely objective reality. Yet how different people perceive that objective reality is dependent on the context they bring to looking at it. Different peoples' subjective evaluation of that completely objective reality can be 180° different.

—

In this case, the dermatologist would say that the hour is a travesty while the March of Dimes volunteer would say it is completely reasonable if not too liberal. The dermatologist might think the regulators and other people responsible for the program are uncaring, uninformed, and perhaps evil. The people in the March of Dimes might think that anyone who opposes a ban on this potent teratogen is uncaring, irresponsible, and perhaps even evil. Neither is evil. Both sides have good intentions and strong, heartfelt reasons for their beliefs. Yet they still see things completely differently.

Not only do they see things completely differently; both sides feel passionately that they are right, and the other side is wrong. Dermatologists passionately fight for their patients with severe acne to have access to this treatment. Dermatologists have seen individuals whose faces have been horribly scarred, scars that isotretinoin could have prevented. Dermatologists have a face to put with the problem. This isn't simply an intellectual exercise to them.

You can probably guess that teratogenicity is a pretty emotional issue to someone who had or knew a child with a severe birth defect. It is not difficult to understand people who feel passionately that birth defects must be prevented.

We don't have to presuppose the world has *good* guys and *bad* guys in order for there to be deep, passionate conflict. We get enough conflict just by having *good* guys and *good* guys. In the abortion debate, people are so at odds, yet their goals are so similar. On the surface, one side sees the other as wanting to promote the killing of human life; the other side sees the other as trying to limit the right of a woman to control her own body, her own life. Neither side seems able to bring themselves to see that the people on the other side are actually good, caring people. The end goals of both sides are probably not as far apart as the conflict suggests. If each side didn't demonize the other, they probably could work together to reduce abortions or perhaps even eliminate the need for abortions without limiting a woman's freedom to control her own body.

Other issues bring out strong emotions. As this book was being written, U.S. armed forces are deployed in Iraq. Some Americans fervently believe that our troops in Iraq will help bring stability, democracy, freedom, and a better life to the Iraqi people. Some Americans fervently believe that having our troops in Iraq hinders progress toward stability, democracy, freedom, and a better life for the Iraqi people. Whichever viewpoint one holds, everyone is hoping and praying that the Iraqis will achieve stability, democracy, freedom, and a better life. In the debate over this war (or occupation, depending on how you perceive it), there are people questioning others' commitment to "funding the troops" or "supporting the troops." These charges elicit strong feelings. Our young people volunteer to serve their country; they put their lives at risk. We should support them. The side that believes the troops are helping Iraq achieve freedom and democracy may feel it is unconscionable not to support the troops' mission. Those that feel that the American presence contributes to instability in Iraq may feel it is unconscionable to waste the lives of brave, young Americans in a counterproductive war. Blaming either side for "not supporting the troops" is wrong. Both sides are truly committed to the welfare of our troops—they just hold different views of how best to assure the welfare of our troops and our nation as a whole.

Our country is full of wonderful people. We have political debates on a wide range of issues. Perhaps it would be more productive if we uniformly recognize that in these debates both sides are well meaning and have good intentions and that disrespecting people on the other side needlessly pushes us farther apart.

—

PART IV

Societal Implications
of Compartments

The Dramatic Impact of Putting People into Compartments

Needless conflict seems to be an automatic result of the organization of people into different compartments. The rivalries between colleges provide a poignant example. I attended college at one of the nerdiest schools on the planet, the University of Chicago. The students' motto for the place was, Where Fun Goes to Die. Our dress was worn jeans and expressive tee shirts (along with the obligatory goose-down coat in the all-too-long winter season). Our idea of entertainment was to attend an evening lecture by one of the faculty along with cheese and cracker snacks. I didn't know it at the time, but life at the University of Chicago in the 1970s was a light-year away from the typical college experience.

I visited Duke University for a medical school interview. What a difference that place was! Every night, there was a party in the main cafeteria, with beer served "on points" from the meal plan. Women wore pretty blouses, skirts, and makeup, things I had never seen women wear at the University of Chicago. Guys at Duke were dressed in buttoned-down shirts and khakis. Compared to the University of Chicago, visiting Duke in 1979 was like going to another planet.

I got to know Duke better during my time at its medical school, and later, nearby University of North Carolina during my dermatology training. The students at these two schools were very, very similar, at least from the context of my University of Chicago background vantage point. Yet the rivalry between people from the two schools was so intense it bordered on the vicious. Grown men, faculty at the schools, would be ecstatic or devastated depending on the outcome of basketball games between the two schools. Try telling them it's just a game.

How is it that the human beings who make up these two schools could be so at odds with each other when they are so similar? Their backgrounds, their cultures, their ethnicity, their future prospects, their educational achievements were nearly identical. Yet their association with their group so defined them that they seemed to think of each other as serious adversaries. One has to wonder just how far we've evolved from pack animals that depend on such associations for their survival.

Grouping people into different compartments can have profound consequences on their relationships. The United States continues to face conflict based on race. No doubt, it has improved greatly over the past decades, culminating in the recent presidential election, but problems still exist. As a student at Duke, I was pleasantly impressed by the easy availability of bathrooms and water fountains in the old hospital building in which my classes were held. It seemed that there were twice as many as a modern building would have. Some of the bathrooms were quite large, others quite small. Then it became clear that there truly were twice as many bathrooms as a building would normally have. The number of bathrooms in the building was a vestige of an earlier time when racial discrimination was more open and systematized.

—

Overt racial discrimination seemed to me so far in the past, yet it really wasn't all that long ago. We are witness to physical evidence of past accepted segregation practices. A generation of people who lived through systematic segregation, people like Betsy Brown, are still with us.

And what was the basis for this discrimination? The color of one's skin. Different human beings are so similar physiologically, yet the color of one's skin might cause a virulent supremacist to think that a person with dark skin was more like a monkey than a human being. Sadly, I've heard such people say as much.

People don't have to be evil to hold discriminatory beliefs; these beliefs are often reinforced by the compartment—by the context—of the observer. Winston-Salem isn't just known for cigarettes. Our town is also home to Old Salem Museum and Gardens (Old Salem 2008). Old Salem is a small community of original buildings, museums, authentic craftsmen practicing their trades, and collections of rare antiques that portray the lives of the Moravian settlement and the diversity of lifestyles that made up the early South. These people struggled with issues of freedom, faith, tradition, government, segregation, and war—issues that remain relevant today.

The Salem part of Winston-Salem was founded in the 1700s by Moravian immigrants. The Moravians were a peace-loving Christian sect that originated in what is the present-day Czech Republic (Moravian Church 2008). Largely pacifists, the Moravians served as conscientious objectors during the Revolutionary War.

The history of the Moravians and their black slaves was recounted in 2006 when the Moravian Church issued a resolution apologizing for its role in slavery (Giunca 2006). Initially, blacks, both freed or enslaved, prayed and lived in Salem with whites in a manner seldom seen in other Southern American towns. But over time that changed. In 1789 the Moravians pushed slaves

—

to the back of the church. Later, blacks were pushed toward the outskirts of town and into churches organized for blacks under white ministers.

The Moravians were not evil people. Far from it, by the standards of their day, they were quite liberal, peace-loving people. Yet today we realize that the discrimination practiced by the Moravian people and their church was completely wrong. Those that discriminated surely didn't see themselves as evil. Their views of the world were shaped by the people around them, by the context of their era.

One doesn't have to go back that far to talk about racism in the United States. In the heart of downtown Winston-Salem is a signpost dedicated to the first sit-in victory in North Carolina. The sign reads,

> On February 8, 1960, Carl Wesley Matthews began the city's sit-in demonstration alone at lunch counters near this site and was soon joined by students from Winston-Salem Teachers College, Atkins High School, and Wake Forest College. The nonviolent protest led to a desegregation agreement signed May 23rd by the City and local businesses. Mr. Matthews, the leader, was the first Black served at a desegregated counter on May 25th. The protest ended in a record 107 days.

Were the people discriminating against blacks in Winston-Salem evil people? It's not hard to view them that way today, but they probably thought they were in the right. They were probably peaceful, churchgoing, G-d-fearing people who were terribly misguided. They lived their lives in their white compartments, and their context permitted them to perceive their discriminatory behavior as good and proper. If you ask Betsy Brown, who grew up in segregated South, she would tell you, "Back then it seemed to us like that was just the way it was."

Perhaps even the appalling apartheid policies of South African whites had a similar basis. Not being a South African, I knew about as much about apartheid as dermatologists knew about their patients' use of their medications. All I knew was that apartheid was a horrible form of discrimination against black and "colored" people, perpetuated by what must have been very evil white South Africans. But a little research on the Internet suggested otherwise.

While outsiders may have seen the Afrikaners as evil racists, many Afrikaners perceived things very differently. For a time, their church, the Dutch Reformed Church, provided moral and religious justification for the apartheid policy (Afrikaner Christianity 2008). One might wonder how a Christian faith could be used to justify apartheid policies. The theology of the Dutch Reformed Church sounds benign, stressing G-d's sovereign control over the universe, the pervasiveness of sinfulness, and Jesus Christ's redemptive work, saving human souls and human culture. This theology led the Dutch Reformed Church to see itself shaping a New Jerusalem in South Africa. While the world saw apartheid and its supporters as evil, Afrikaners reportedly saw themselves as the obedient people of G-d, shaping a society according to biblical Christian principles.

The Afrikaners saw strong parallels between themselves as the people of G-d and the biblical nation of Israel as the people of G-d. In striking similarity to my Jewish heritage, Afrikaners saw themselves as an embattled minority struggling to be obedient to G-d while confronted with hostile forces all around. Their feeling of attachment to the land of South Africa was little different from our Jewish attachment to Jerusalem and Israel. The sense of threat, from the black majority and the outside world, may have

---

contributed to the church's support of apartheid policies. While the outside world saw Afrikaners as evil oppressors, the Afrikaners may have seen themselves as oppressed, G-d-loving people. This more benign understanding of white South Africans contrasted so deeply with the general impression people held of apartheid and its proponents that firsthand confirmation seemed in order. We turn to Dr. Alan Menter, a Dallas dermatologist, to tell us more.

Alan Menter is a dermatology hero. Alan has special expertise in the treatment of psoriasis. Other dermatologists send him their most difficult and complicated patients. Alan is a caring physician loved by his patients. He has done critical work on how to best use psoriasis treatments, on the development of new psoriasis treatments, and on the basic genetic cause of psoriasis. He has been active in teaching psoriasis management to dermatologists all over the United States. Alan's greatest contribution to dermatology, however, has been his unyielding commitment to advocacy for patients with psoriasis. He founded the International Psoriasis Council, a global nonprofit organization dedicated to advancing psoriasis research and treatment. The International Psoriasis Council has begun to mobilize and coordinate the efforts of leading dermatologists all over the globe to advance psoriasis research and treatment.

Dermatology is a niche of medicine that has attracted many interesting people, but Alan's story is among the most interesting I have encountered (Menter 2003). Martin Alan Menter was born in Yorkshire, England, in 1941. His father was South African, had gone to Dublin to study medicine, and met Alan's Irish Jewish mother there. One of Alan's earliest memories is of taking a mail boat, from Southampton, England, to Cape Town, South Africa, in 1946 after the end of the war.

Alan grew up in Johannesburg, part of a liberal family by South African standards. His father did a tremendous amount of work in the black community, starting the first clinic to deliver black babies in the compounds of Johannesburg, something that wasn't allowed by the government. His father used a double-decker bus as a clinic. Alan would accompany his father to see patients in the clinic on nights and weekends. At home, Alan's father was demanding, both of scholarly and sporting activities. Alan's sporting focus was rugby. His father would spend hours working with Alan on his rugby kicking skills. Rugby is a theme that runs through Alan's life and the lives of South African people.

The Menter home life recognized some British traditions, particularly around mealtime. The family was Jewish, regularly attending services on high holidays. There were Saturday visits to the synagogue as well, but Alan's passion was for sports, not religion, and he would leave the synagogue as quickly as possible and head to the rugby fields.

Alan attended an all-boys public school run by the government. There were also truly excellent British private schools to which the English gentry sent their children, but the Menter family was not elitist. Alan considered himself very fortunate. "Because of the apartheid system, most of the money was put into white education," he said. "The poor blacks had to make do with what was left. We had wonderful facilities, including wonderful sporting facilities and big playing fields. Even though this was an English school, the government put a lot of energy into it. When I went to school from 1946 through 1958, twelve years of schooling, it was still very much a British kind of tradition even though the Afrikaners had come into power in 1948." The Afrikaner government had created parallel school systems. "Right across the road from our English high school was an Afrikaans high school. We never met those kids except when we played rugby against them once a year. It was like two separate worlds." Within the English schools, students learned British history. In the Afrikaner schools, students learned Afrikaner history. The apartheid system didn't just separate whites from blacks; it also separated the Afrikaners of Dutch ancestry from the English speakers of British ancestry.

For college and medical school, Alan attended the University of Witwatersrand in Johannesburg, an Oxford-type university by South African standards. Witwatersrand is a Dutch name meaning the white water's reef, and the university was surrounded by gold mines. "Even though we had this tragic apartheid system in South Africa, the medical school and our university were a bastion of 'liberalism.' The apartheid government would try to shut us down all the time because we admitted people of all races and color," Alan said. "Two of the students who dissected with me were nonwhite. I used to go with one of them, Benson Nghona, back to the black area where he lived. He was not allowed to live in the white area. It was very unusual for whites to go to black areas because they were totally separate. We became close friends."

Because of rugby, Alan did not get involved in the protest movement. There was some violence, but it wasn't black-white violence, it was Afrikaner English violence. The Afrikaners felt the English were going against the law of the land, which was apartheid. "We 'flouted' those laws by allowing black students on our campus."

Alan had a broad medical experience, serving patients in both white and black hospitals. In addition to the rigors and fun of medical school, Alan had a rugby career. He served as captain of the university rugby team. "When I graduated from the under-19 juniors into the university team, I was made captain, the youngest-ever university captain. I played rugby throughout the six years of medical school. The collegiality of rugby and cricket, the Saturday night parties with beer drinking, and the rigors of medical school made it a busy, exciting, wonderful time."

Alan moved from Witwaterstrand to the medical school in Pretoria for his dermatology training. Pretoria was the seat of Afrikaner power. He describes it as a lily-white place and a very religious place. The South African government was based in Pretoria. Alan had to learn Afrikaans to communicate there, having learned only a little as a second language in high school. The culture shift was considerable. Worst of all, he had to leave his beloved rugby team at Witwatersrand behind.

Shortly after arriving in Pretoria, however, Alan was asked to join the University of Pretoria rugby team and fill in for an injured player. Alan now lives in Texas and says going from Witwatersrand to Pretoria was like going from the University of Texas football team to the one at the University of Oklahoma—he was joining the enemy. Playing against Pretoria had been the Witwatersrand team's big game every year. Somewhat reluctant, he played, and he played well. He moved up. He became team captain, the first Jewish team captain in their history. Eventually, he even played on the South African national team, donning the green-and-gold jersey that defined the team. He took a one-month absence from his new dermatology job, his wife, and their four-month old baby to represent South Africa in the international rugby tournament in France.

Rugby was the traditional Afrikaner white sport; it was a second religion to them. "The Afrikaners looked upon rugby as their way of showing the rest of the world that they could compete even though they had created this dreadful apartheid system," Alan said. It was through rugby that Alan really got to know these "evil" Afrikaners. He met them after they attended church, when they came out to play rugby. He partied with them, and he drank a lot of beer with them. He had the chance to see them as they were and as they saw themselves.

Despite the despicable apartheid system they had created, Alan found that Afrikaners were peace oriented, generally loving, family-oriented people who were brought up to believe they had been oppressed by the British, owed by the Bible, and willed by G-d to create a white culture in South Africa. The Afrikaner owned a history of religious persecution in Europe, of oppression by the British in South Africa, of being a minority outnumbered by violent others. The Afrikaners' Christian faith did indeed support the development and perpetuation of apartheid.

One of Alan's Afrikaner rugby teammates was Dawie de Villiers, one of rugby's greatest scrum halves and captain of the South African national team from 1965 to 1970. Dawie was religious, descended from French Huguenots (another persecuted religious group that had sought refuge in South Africa), and like Southern Baptists and other very religious Afrikaners, he didn't drink. Alan asked Dawie when there would be a black prime minister—he answered rather ominously in Afrikaans, "*Nooit in my lewe*" (never in my lifetime). Good, religious Afrikaners could not and did not see evil in the apartheid system.

But the apartheid system did end, and it was the Afrikaners themselves who ended it. The sports boycott against South Africa, against their beloved rugby, played a major role. Mandela also played a major role, giving people a vision of the future in which white South Africans would still be involved. When Mandela came into power, Dawie de Villiers was named to the cabinet, minister of sport. He became part of the black establishment.

Alan Menter believes that Mandela, the black president of South Africa, sealed the end of apartheid in 1995. The blacks had hated rugby. They saw the green-and-gold jersey of the South African rugby team as a hated symbol of apartheid. After apartheid ended, the international rugby tournament was held in South Africa, and the South African team was victorious. Mandela went on the field and heartily congratulated the South African team; he wore the green-and-gold uniform that black South Africans had learned to hate. This expression of unity left people in tears. Mandela was prepared to forgive both twenty-seven years of imprisonment and the apartheid system.

The Afrikaners were warm, lovely, great people, but like others, they were not immune from making huge misjudgments. They saw themselves as peaceful, oppressed people while the world saw them as evil for their system of apartheid. Alan lived with them, played with them, and got drunk with them. He got to know them as they saw themselves. Alan said, "The interesting thing is the Dutch have been the nicest, most liberal people. They and the Afrikaners went into totally different directions. Descended from the same people, environment, and circumstances took them in totally different directions."

With the end of apartheid, people who had hated each other grew to integrate. There are still vestiges of hate and black insecurity about how South African commerce is controlled, but the situation is slowly improving. Nevertheless, there are still places, in South Africa and elsewhere, where people don't want to be integrated. There are still some Afrikaners who continue to fear that the black South African historically tribal-based people are an inherently warring, violent people.

As far as people have come toward recognizing human equality, we still have a tendency to group people and see them as different, despite the fact that our similarities far outweigh our differences. Consider Judaism and Islam. The two religions worship the same deity. Both pride themselves on their monotheistic beliefs. The basic tenets of the religions—truth, justice, and peace for Judaism and peace while living in accordance with G-d's will for Islam—are basically the same. Yet there is sharp tension between the groups. The physiologies of Israeli Jews and Palestinian Arabs

—

are entirely identical. Culturally, the similarities between the two far outweigh their differences. Yet many people believe that Israelis and Palestinians can't possibly coexist, despite the fact that a significant proportion of Israel's population is Palestinian and that they already peacefully coexist. There are people who look at Israel and see its treatment of Palestinians as similar to South African apartheid. On the other side are people who feel that the Israeli Jew is the one who is oppressed. The topic is at the heart of much conflict in the world and deserving of more attention.

The Israeli Palestinian Conflict (Part I): Where We Are Now

The issues we currently face in the Israeli Palestinian conflict are beautifully laid out in two commentaries, one by Cal Thomas and the other by Paul Craig Roberts, both published the very same day, January 17, 2008. Thomas's article, "Misplaced Faith," chides former President Bush for fantasizing when Bush proposed that peace between Israelis and Palestinians is possible (Thomas 2008). Thomas stated that all the many previous attempts to persuade the "Jewish lamb to lie down with the Arab lion" have failed, and any new one is also bound to fail despite whatever pressure is put on Israel "to do more." Thomas shows how the impasse is entirely the fault of Palestinians, pointing out that even while Bush was talking about peace, Palestinian organizations were calling for liberation of Israeli cities that do not figure in the debate over Israeli "occupation" [Thomas's quotes] of Palestinian land. Thomas fingered the Palestinian government for failing to comply with even a single agreement: failing to cease terror, failing to cease the incitement of violence against Jews, failing to reform textbooks teaching hatred of Jews and Christians, and failing to limit the number of Palestinian police permitted to carry weapons.

Thomas makes clear that Israeli concessions are useless. "If, after all of Israel's concessions, her enemies have failed to take a single step toward peace, what makes anyone think that more concessions will turn a one-way street into a two-lane thoroughfare?" he asks. "The best that can be expected from the Palestinian side is a temporary lull in the violence followed by the creation of a pretext for more violence and demands for new concessions." Thomas sees an American push for peace as only making things worse for Israel as the other side is committed "to be free of our freedom and impose Sharia law on all."

Cal Thomas doesn't mince words. Neither does Paul Craig Roberts. Roberts's article, "Bringing Death and Destruction to Muslims," offered a radically different view of the conflict (Roberts 2008):

> Hezbollah and Hamas are two organizations that exist because of Israeli aggression against Palestine and Lebanon. The two organizations are branded "terrorist" because they resist Israel's theft of Palestine and Israel's designs on southern Lebanon. Both organizations are resistance organizations. They resist Israel's territorial expansion and this makes them "terrorist." They are terrorists because they don't receive billions in US military aid and cannot put armies in the field with tanks, fighter jets and helicopter gunships, backed up by US spy satellites and Israel's nuclear weapons . . . . However, Palestine is so thoroughly under the Israeli heel that Hamas can resist only with suicide bombers and obsolete rockets. It is dishonest to damn the terrorist response but not the policies that provoke the response . . . Israel, protected by the US, has disobeyed UN resolutions for four decades and has been methodically squeezing

Palestinians out of Palestine. Americans do not think of themselves or of Israel as terrorist states, but the evidence is complete and overwhelming. Thanks to the power of the Israel Lobby, Americans only know the Israeli side of the story, which is that evil anti-semite Palestinians will not let blameless Israelis live in peace and persist in their unjustified terror attacks on an innocent Israeli state . . . Americans don't know what terror is. To know terror, you have to be a Palestinian, an Iraqi, or an Afghan . . . Terror is families attending a wedding being blown to pieces by an American missile or bomb and the survivors being blown to pieces at the funeral of the newlyweds. Terror is troops breaking down your door in the middle of the night, putting guns to your heads, and carrying off brothers, sons, and husbands with bags over their heads and returning to rape the unprotected women. Terror is being waterboarded in one of America's torture dungeons. Terror is "when you run from hospital ward to hospital ward, from prison to prison, from militia to militia looking for your loved one only to recognize them from their teeth fillings in some morgue." For people targeted by American hegemony, terror is realizing that Americans have no moral conscience. In the . . . minds of the White House . . . the massive deaths for which America is responsible, including those inflicted by Israel, have nothing to do with Muslim enmity toward America. Instead, Muslims hate us for our "freedom and democracy."

What is the Israeli Palestinian conflict all about? Is it, as someone with Cal Thomas's perspective might say, the story of the oppressed Jewish people, a lamb, under constant attack, facing unrelenting hatred from evil Muslim nations? Or is the conflict a story more like the one told by Roberts, the story of the mighty nation Israel, backed by America, the world's only superpower, mercilessly dispossessing and terrorizing the oppressed Palestinian people?

Both Cal Thomas and Paul Craig Roberts have impressive resumes. Cal Thomas was born in Washington, DC, in 1942 and attended American University (Wikipedia, Cal Thomas, 2008). During the 1960s and early 1970s, he worked as a reporter at NBC News. He has written ten books, writes a syndicated column appearing in hundreds of newspapers, and is an award-winning TV talk show participant. Thomas was also vice president of the Moral Majority from 1980 to 1985. Paul Craig Roberts went to college at the Georgia Institute of Technology, received a PhD from the University of Virginia, and studied at the University of California, Berkeley, and Oxford University (Wikipedia, Paul Craig Roberts 2008). He is a former editor and columnist for the *Wall Street Journal, Business Week*, and Scripps Howard News Service. Roberts was John M. Olin Fellow at the Institute for Political Economy, Senior Research Fellow at the Hoover Institution, Stanford University, and was Distinguished Fellow at the Cato Institute from 1993 to 1996. He served as an assistant secretary of the treasury in the Reagan administration earning fame as the Father of Reaganomics.

The vast differences between the two stories Cal Thomas and Paul Craig Roberts tell of the Israeli Palestine conflict is not because one of the writers is brilliant and the other is an idiot. Like dermatologists' and March of Dimes volunteers' views on isotretinoin, and like the differences between how Afrikaners viewed themselves versus how they were viewed by the world, well meaning, caring, intelligent people on each side of the debate look at the same objective facts and construct two completely different perceptions of reality.

Israelis kill Palestinians, and Palestinians kill Israelis. Israelis kill Palestinians with some of the most advanced weaponry the world has ever seen, including F-16 fighter jets and Apache helicopters built and funded by the United States. Palestinians kill Israelis with low-tech bombs, sometimes carried by suicide bombers, and rockets. Either way, there is a clear, unarguable objective reality: people die.

What do people perceive when these people are killed? When an Israeli Jew is killed by a Palestinian suicide bomber, Israelis perceive terrorism. Many Palestinians, however, may perceive the killing as retaliation. When Israelis strike back with F-16 fighter jets and blow up an apartment building, Israelis call it retaliation while Palestinians perceive the killing as terrorism. Killing is the objective reality.

Context	Israeli Kills People	Palestinian Kills People
Palestinians were expelled from their homes	Terrorism	Retaliation
Jews returned to their homeland	Retaliation	Terrorism

Whether the killing is called terrorism or retaliation is not a function of how the killing was done or even of who was killed. It is a function of the context of the observer. Many of us look at suicide bombing and see something completely different, something far more horrific, than a nameless bomb dropped by a heroic pilot flying an F-16. But Carnegie's golden rule tells us the mother, family, friends, and people of the child killed by the F-16 probably see using an F-16 against totally defenseless people to be utterly inhumane, uncivilized terrorism. They may see the lone bomber, fighting back against the militarily superior enemy, as a hero.

To tell people whose loved one was killed that the killing wasn't terrorism won't be believed. It doesn't matter whether the killing was done with a crude rocket or a laser-guided missile. The parents, friends, and people of the dead will see what was done as a terrorist act. When their side responds with violence, they will view what they did as retaliation.[5] As we saw with the perceptions of the darkness of the black-and-white letters in a visual illusion or the apparent blue color of a vein that we know is not blue, the brain's perceptions may be uncontrollably strong and not easily changed by logical arguments or objective proof. Each side quite

---

[5.] Even though the Palestinians kill far fewer Israelis than the Israelis kill Palestinians, many Americans perceive that the actions of the "terrorist" Palestinians are much worse because of their "intent." Americans perceive that the "intent" of the terrorists is to kill civilians, while Israeli's intent is to achieve peace. On the other hand, Palestinians perceive the intent of the killers as to stop the violence Israel commits and to help Palestinians return to their homes; Palestinians perceive that the intent of the killing Israel does is to keep Palestinians from returning to their homes without any compunction for the death of Palestinian civilians. Perceived "intent" is probably less important than we make it out to be. Had the terrorists who committed the destruction of 9-11 jumped safely from the planes just before impact, they would not have been suicide bombers, but it would not have lessened the horror of what they had done in any way. If a Palestinian terrorist were to steal an Israeli jet and "accidently" miss while trying to bomb the headquarters of the Israeli Defense Force or the office of the Israeli Prime Minister—killing large numbers of Jewish men, women and children in the adjacent neighborhood in the process—no one in Israel would promote giving that Palestinian a hero's medal of honor for his or her intent not to kill civilians.

146

definitively sees what the other side does as criminally wrong and what their own side does as excusable redress. With killing that has gone back and forth for so long, over sixty years, each side sees itself as a victim and the other side as an instigator.

The United States is more than a bystander in the conflict. We call Iran a terrorist nation because Iran has provided support to people we consider terrorists. It isn't hard to figure how the Unites States looks to the Muslim world when Muslims see Israel kill Palestinians or destroy the Lebanese infrastructure with U.S. support.

The context in which people view the Israeli Palestinian conflict is intensely emotional. My grandparents had parents, brothers, sisters, extended family, and friends killed by the Nazis in Europe. It grieves my parents just to think about how their family members were killed. Hearing a car door slam may evoke memories of the train cars that took family members to the concentration camps. There is no question that Jews who survived this see themselves as victims. They are terrified that it could happen again. The horror they survived is their context, and it profoundly affects how they perceive events in Israel's history and events that occur today.

To have some idea of the depth of emotion that pervades this conflict, one has to put a face on it. We can know that there are 40,000 Americans killed each year in auto accidents, yet it doesn't affect us nearly as much as reading in a local paper about a particular child who was killed. We can know that 40,000 women die of breast cancer each year, but it doesn't move us as does breast cancer in one of our friends or loved ones. In the case of the Israeli Palestinian conflict, one such face that moved us was that of Gilad Shalit, an Israeli soldier who was captured by Palestinians on June 25, 2006 (Wikipedia, Gilad Shalit, 2008). The entire Jewish world was shaken by his being abducted and held hostage (while some Palestinians viewed it as his being "taken prisoner" rather than "held hostage"). Pictures of him and his family were circulated. The Israeli Defense Force launched an offensive into Gaza in response. There was palpable horror in the taking of this one Israeli by Palestinians.

Once one has truly felt the horror felt by the family, friends, and people of Gilad Shalit, one can probably begin to understand what the Palestinians feel. For each Israeli Gilad Shalit taken by the enemy, there are hundreds, if not thousands, of Palestinian Gilad Shalit's taken hostage (some Israelis would call it "taken prisoner") by the Israelis. From our perspective, it may not seem so horrible to take so many nameless people prisoner, much as 40,000 automobile deaths each year don't intrude on our daily consciousness. But on the other side, each prisoner is a human being; they have families, friends, and other loved ones. We can understand the horror Palestinians feel because we know what horror we feel when it is one of our own.

With isotretinoin, we saw how good people can look at one objective reality and perceive totally different things. The emotional baggage of the Holocaust and the displacement of hundreds of thousands of Palestinians affect people's perceptions of the objective reality of the Israeli Palestinian conflict, a reality in which people are being killed. One side may perceive the blowing up a bus or a disco as justified retaliation; the other side may perceive the isolation of Gaza and the killing of far greater numbers of Palestinian with tanks and F-16s as justified retaliation. The objective reality remains the same: people are dying.

—

The Israeli Palestinian Conflict (Part II): How We Got Here

The Israeli Palestinian conflict has largely become a tit for tat, violence for violence, circular conflict. If we are ever to figure out how to end this conflict, we need to understand what got us here and how it is perceived by both sides of the conflict. Knowing how compartments complicate our ability to make accurate judgments, it's clear that objectively understanding the root causes of the Israeli Palestinian conflict will be difficult. It was difficult to see how patients used their medications until there were electronic monitors. It is difficult to know exactly what happened that generated the Israeli Palestinian conflict we see today.

All three principles of compartments affect our understanding of the conflict. Within our compartment, there are some things we just don't see, others that we see that aren't representative, and still others that are representative but that may be viewed very differently depending on the context brought by the observer.

I have been told, and told passionately, that the heart of this conflict is a conflict between peaceful religions like Judaism and Christianity and a violent religion seeking world domination, Islam. My Jewish and Christian friends point to the Jewish holy book teaching peace while the Islamic holy book teaches violence. This is the common error of believing a misrepresentative selection from the other compartment. Ask a Muslim about the Koran, and they will tell you it is a book that teaches peace. Listen to many Jews talk about the Koran, and they will pick out a passage they say proves Islam is violent. Yet it would not be hard to look in the Jewish holy books and pull out single passages that make Judaism look violent. Any Jew would tell you such passages are not representative of our faith.

It may seem to us that Islam seeks to dominate the world, despite Muslims claims to the contrary. But if we think Islam is trying to dominate the world, imagine how it looks to Muslims when they see that the largely Christian United States has its armed forces all over the globe, that Christians are sent as missionaries to every corner of the planet, and that Christians support the taking of Palestine from Palestinian Muslims who used to live there.

We know our religion is peaceful. We know we aren't seeking world domination. We wish we didn't have to police the world, though we feel obligated to do so at times. But to Muslims, it would be hard to know that's what we're feeling. The Muslim religion isn't particularly violent or evil either. The Muslims are not seeking world domination. But to us, it's hard to see that. A cosmic clash of religions doesn't seem to be the heart of Israeli Palestinian conflict.

One of the root differences in how the two sides view the conflict seems to be in how they mentally construct the founding of Israel. Was Israel founded as a "Jewish state" as we tend to frame it, or was it founded as a "Jewish state at the expense of Palestinians already living there"? Growing up Jewish in Washington, DC, attending Hebrew school, I was taught that Jews came to an empty land of deserts and swamps and a few nomadic Arabs. We were proud that we drained the swamps, planted trees, developed farms, and created the great country of Israel, and we were taught that Arabs hated us out of jealousy of our success. We weren't told and didn't see, however, that there were hundreds of thousands of Palestinians already living in Palestine before we arrived. In 1914, after immigration of European Jews to Palestine had already begun, Palestine had an estimated 657,000 Muslim inhabitants, 70,000 Christians, and 59,000 Jews (Morris, 2001; p. 83). Palestine wasn't empty swamps and deserts. Had the herd mentality of our compartment not gotten the best of us, we might have figured out that the land couldn't have been just deserts and swamps if there were 700,000 refugees displaced by the creation of Israel.

Growing up in the Jewish community, what we saw of Arabs was uniformly bad, and what we saw of ourselves was uniformly good. Arabs hated us, we were taught. Any stories we read about Arabs had to do with war and killing and hatred. Of course we didn't see the day-to-day lives of any of the far greater number of Arabs and Muslims who were living peaceful lives—none of them were newsworthy. When we looked at ourselves, almost all we saw were the day-to-day peaceful lives, G-d-fearing people, praying for peace, praying that our enemies would eventually leave us alone. We heard horrific stories of attacks on Jews: perhaps the worst was the story of the 1929 massacre of Jews in Hebron, a mass murder of over sixty Jews, including a dozen women and three children under the age of three (Wikipedia, 1929 Hebron Massacre, 2008). On the other hand, we didn't spend much time learning about how scores of Arabs were also killed in the 1929 riots or about how Jewish terrorists were the first to plant bombs in buses and crowded civilian markets in Palestine (Morris 2001, p. 147).

The quiet times, the normal times, the usual times, when hundreds of thousands of Palestinian Muslims lived peacefully together with tens of thousands of Christians and tens of thousands of Jews were completely invisible, probably not taught or studied by either side in this great conflict. The Hebron massacres (one in 1929, the other in 1994) stand out, like postal worker violent rage; this is what comes to mind when people think or talk about the people on the other side of the conflict. The normal, friendly human interactions that took place on a day-to-day basis were the true background and, like the steady drone of an air conditioner, were never heard. The Hebron massacres, the intermittent violent events, like the sudden change in sound when an air conditioner cuts off, grabbed people's attention.

One of the pillars of the justification for Israel we were taught is that we Jews came to Israel looking to live at peace with the Palestinians and that the problem was the Arabs' unwillingness to live with us. We learned how, at the start of the war of 1948 that created Israel, Zionist Jews begged Palestinians to stay and not run away. We learned that the Palestinians fled at the behest of Arab countries so the Arabs could wipe out the Jews.[6] What we weren't taught was the Zionists' military plans included Haganah Plan D, the text of which described destruction of entire Arab villages.

A Jewish dermatologist sent me information he had on the Israeli Palestine conflict. One of the items was a history of the Israel Palestine conflict that included a mention of Plan D (Middle East Web, Israel and Palestine, 2008). The document he sent stated, Plan D "envisioned the 'temporary' evacuation of Arab civilians from towns in certain strategic areas." The actual text of Plan D describes, "Destruction of villages" (setting fire to, blowing up, and

---

[6.]   Even if Palestinian families had fled their homes for safety because Arab armies were coming, those families should have been allowed to return to their homes when the hostilities had ended. They weren't allowed to return, not because they were violent people, but simply because they weren't Jewish. One doesn't have to be Muslim to perceive the inequity.

planting mines in the debris) and "the population must be expelled outside the borders of the state" (Middle East Web, Plan Dalet, 2008). It would be a stretch to perceive that destruction of entire villages and planting mines in the debris represents "temporary evacuation." A Saudi dermatologist explained to me that she was taught that the Zionists drove out Arab inhabitants and set villages on fire. That understanding of history doesn't seem too far from the actual wording of Plan D. In his book, *The Iron Wall*, Avi Shlaim describes it as follows (Shlaim 2001, p. 31):

> Although the wording of Plan D was vague, its objective was to clear the interior of the country of hostile and potentially hostile Arab elements, and in this sense it provided a warrant for expelling civilians. By implementing Plan D in April and May, the Haganah [the precursor to the Israeli Defense Force] thus directly and decisively contributed to the birth of the Palestinian refugee problem . . . Palestinian society disintegrated under the impact of the Jewish military offensive that got under way in April, and the exodus of the Palestinians was set in motion. There were many reasons for the Palestinian exodus, including the early departure of the Palestinian leaders when the going got tough, but the most important reason was Jewish military pressure. Plan D was not a political blueprint for the expulsion of Palestine's Arabs: it was a military plan with military and territorial objectives. However, by ordering the capture of Arab cities and the destruction of villages, it both permitted and justified the forcible expulsion of Arab civilians. By the end of 1948 the number of Palestinian refugees had swollen to around 700,000. But the first and largest wave of refugees occurred before the official outbreak of hostilities on 15 May.

The historical documentation offered in Plan D suggests Jews did play an important role in the violent displacement of 700,000 Palestinian men, women, and children. Israeli historian Benny Morris (2004) described the 1948 expulsions of Palestinians in the Israeli newspaper *Ha'aretz*:

> Based on many documents that were not available to me when I wrote the original book, most of them from the Israel Defense Forces Archives. What the new material shows is that there were far more Israeli acts of massacre than I had previously thought. To my surprise, there were also many cases of rape. In the months of April-May 1948, units of the Haganah [the pre-state defense force that was the precursor of the IDF] were given operational orders that stated explicitly that they were to uproot the villagers, expel them and destroy the villages themselves.

The discovery of Plan D documents showed that the Palestinians were expelled and their villages destroyed and mined to keep them from returning. Still, an observer whose context is the absolute righteousness of the state of Israel and the unconditional necessity of a home for the Jewish people can observe the wording of Plan D and still honestly believe that the Zionists committed no crime. Such observers also may think those who say the Zionists did commit crimes must be "anti-Semitic," even when such comments are made by Jews who seek peace and justice for both Jews and Muslims alike.

Author Ali Abunimah commented on the effect of the Jewish history, the Jewish context, on this very issue (Abunimah 2006):

> The question of how the Palestinians came to be in exile has always been at the center of any argument over the legitimacy of Israel. To Israelis and most Jews, the

Jewish State is a miracle that represents redemption from the unspeakable horrors of the Nazi Holocaust. Israel is an emotional insurance policy against the visceral vulnerability that many Jews still feel, a vulnerability born of centuries of persecution in Europe. Israel is a touchstone of identity and a rallying point for community. The notion that its creation was achieved with the blood and suffering of others, that bad deeds were done and continue to be done, is unbearable emotionally and threatening politically. *It can't have been*, they say, *therefore, it wasn't.*

We don't have electronic monitors to tell us what really happened in 1948. Did Jews try to live with Palestinians or try to displace them? In a letter to the *University of Chicago Magazine*, John Mearshimer (author of *The Israel Lobby*) wrote, "Jews had come to Palestine to create a Jewish state, which meant that they had to take the Palestinians' land away from them. How else could you create a Jewish state in a land filled with Palestinians" (Mearshimer 2006)? Mearshimer's point is simple and clear, though depending on context, one might see otherwise. Many Jews still believe that Arabs started the conflict, even though the Zionist Jews came to Palestine with the goal of creating a state for themselves in a land that was already populated by hundreds of thousands of people. Israel's founding father, David Ben-Gurion said in 1919, "There is a gulf, and nothing can bridge it . . . I do not know what Arab will agree that Palestine should belong to the Jews . . . . We, as a nation, want this country to be ours"(Morris 2001, p. 91). Ben-Gurion reiterated the point in 1936, saying, "There is a great conflict. We and they want the same thing: We both want Palestine. And that is the fundamental conflict." In his book, *Righteous Victims: A History of the Zionist-Arab Conflict 1881-2001*,

Morris claims Ben-Gurion's ultimate goal was taking the entire country (Morris 2001, p. 138):

> [A] Jewish state in part [of Palestine] is not an end, but a beginning . . . . Our possession is important not only for itself . . . through this we increase our power, and every increase in power facilitates getting hold of the country in its entirety. Establishing a [small] state . . . will serve as a very potent lever in our historical efforts to redeem the whole country.

Morris goes on to suggest that Ben-Gurion saw nothing immoral in compulsory expulsion of Palestinians (Morris 2001, p. 144). It seems likely that Ben-Gurion and Zionists did play a major role in creating the Palestinian refugee problem. It would be nice to believe the stories that Jews returned to a homeland that was for practical purposes devoid of other people, that it was just swamps and deserts that nobody cared about, that the few Palestinians who were living there left in order to try to further the killing of Jews, and that part of the Muslim religion is to kill Jews, but none of those stories seems to be true. The truth seems to be that there were human beings—men, women, and children—living peacefully in Palestine, that Jews who were treated horribly in Europe felt the need to create a country of their own, and that it hardly mattered to them that Palestinian Arabs were already living there. Jews felt their actions were justified by their perceived need for security, and in treating Palestinians as they did (and continue to do), they created widespread hatred of Israel (and perhaps of Jews too) in the Muslim world.

Muslims should know that the Christians and Jews who give Israel unconditional support are not evil people. Far from it, Christians and Jews are good, caring people who believe in justice.

We can understand why supporters of Israel feel as they do based on the experiences they have observed and based on what their teachers taught them, including the horrors of the Holocaust and terrorist killings of Jews. The stories Christians and Jews are told largely ignore the role Jews played in displacing Palestinians. The support for Israel does not come from malevolence against Palestinians. In fact, it truly pains supporters of Israel to see Palestinians suffer. There is no evil conspiracy among Israel's supporters, Jewish or Christian, to control America or to kill Muslims.

Similarly, we should be able to see that Muslims who call for Israel to be removed from the map are not evil people either. Their perceptions are also based on their observations of the conflict. They saw the violent displacement of Palestinians and the continued violence against them. Muslims are also pained by the horrors of the Holocaust and have no desire to see Jews killed. When Muslims say Israel (or the "Zionist entity") must be removed from the map, they refer to letting Palestinians return to their homes, not the wholesale slaughter of Jews.

A Syrian dermatopathologist colleague, Dr. Sate Hamza, participated in an online discussion of Israeli Palestinian issues with a Jewish dermatology colleague and ended with the following comment:

> We are disagreeing regarding issues but it is obvious to me that we both have something essential in common and that is a desire to reach a peaceful and just resolution for this intractable conflict.

As far apart as both sides are in the Israeli Palestinian conflict, they share the common goals of seeking peace and justice.

The Israeli Palestinian Conflict (Part III): Where Can We Go from Here

It's not hard to imagine how the views of Arabs have been shaped. Do they grow up seeing Jews praying for peace on a day-to-day basis? Not likely. On the other hand, do they notice when our side kills a Palestinian Muslim? Of course they do. While my upbringing taught me to see only the worst in Arabs and Muslims, I have little doubt that their upbringing would be equally misleading about Israelis and other Jews. Misperceptions of each other need to change.

Single passages from the Torah or the Koran don't tell us what their religions are like; people's behavior does. It is so *obvious* to us that Muslim behavior is violent. We see the terrorism they commit. We are told the only thing such people understand is violence, so we must be violent in return. We are told that terrorists are evil, and that giving in to their demands—appeasement—will only encourage more terrorism. However, if we accept this as a universal law of human behavior, the symmetry of Carnegie's golden rule tells us the Muslim side is probably saying the same thing about us.

It shouldn't be hard to believe that well meaning, caring, G-d-fearing, otherwise peaceful Muslim people see our troops in Middle East countries, our support for Israel's killing of Palestinians, and our support for dictators (along with our hypocritical rejection of democratically elected leaders we don't like) and think that the violence we commit is terrorism. They would think that the only thing people like us understand is violence and, therefore, they must be violent in return. Zacarias Moussaoui so much as told us so.

Answering the violence we face with more violence will beget more violence in return. There is another way. We can treat others as we would want to be treated. The Cal Thomases say that this wouldn't work, that we've tried "compromise," and it has gotten us nowhere. From the Muslim perspective, perhaps they don't think we've begun to compromise. They see that hundreds of thousands of Palestinian men, women, and children were made refugees by the war that created Israel and that those refugees have not been permitted to return to rebuild their homes and villages and lives.

Some have compared what Israel has done to Palestinians to the Holocaust the Jews faced. With a background like mine, you don't throw the word "Holocaust" around lightly. My family came from Poland, and many of them were murdered there. I'm not comfortable calling what was done to Palestinian people another Holocaust. The comparison doesn't seem to fit. Six million Palestinians were not killed in gas chambers.

That said, one shouldn't minimize the horrors that were done to Palestinians. Some 700,000 Palestinian men, women, and children were made refugees in the violence that created the state of Israel. Their villages were destroyed. To hear an Israeli leader say as Golda Meir said, "There are no Palestinians," makes me sad; I'm sure it makes Palestinians feel angry. For Jews to believe there are no Palestinian people is simply a misconception common to one compartment. Benny Morris's book, *Righteous Victims: A History of the Zionist-Arab Conflict, 1881-1999,* describes a 1905 meeting of Zionists in Basel at which a Palestinian Jew, Yitzhak Epstein said, "There is one question which is equal to all others: the question of our relations with the Arabs . . . We have forgotten one small matter: There is in our beloved land an entire nation, which has occupied it for hundreds of years and has never thought to leave it"(2001, p. 57). The early Zionists recognized that there were already Arabs in Palestine and that they would have to be displaced to create a Jewish state. To ignore the injustice done to Palestinians in the creation of the Jewish state is not consistent with the morals of Jewish upbringing.

Ignoring the injustice is also counterproductive. Palestinian anger is stoked by living in refugee camps, knowing their homes and villages had been destroyed by the Israelis. It should not be surprising some feel like throwing the Jews out, perhaps killing them if necessary. Yet, if the Israelis apologized and offered Palestinians the chance to return and help to rebuild, there would be no reason to continue the hatred. People are forgiving, especially if they have the economic incentive to forgive. Just as the United States and Vietnam forge friendly relations today, offering the Palestinians the right to return would be a major step toward a true peace for both sides.[7] Can the

---

7.   Some would argue that the responsibility for the Palestinian refugees should fall on the Arab states because Jews fled Arab states after Israel had been created. Giving the homes of Palestinians to Jews from Europe, Russia or even Arab countries does not compensate Palestinian men, women and children who had been expelled from their homes and villages by the Jews. There was no reciprocal "population transfer" between the European Jews who created Israel and the Palestinians who the Jews replaced.

United States stop its support of Israel's military and instead support Israel by offering to help in the repatriation of Palestinian refugees? We can, and we should.

The major objection to doing so is that it would mean the destruction of Israel. The "destruction of Israel" means different things to different people. At best, it means that Israel is no longer a homeland run by and for Jews. Some people find that possibility unthinkable. From an American perspective, based on our principles of freedom and equality, a democratic state that gives equal rights to all people regardless of their religion is not a horrible outcome. From a moral American Jewish perspective, this would be a laudable outcome.

With the context of the Holocaust still fresh in some people's minds, however, many perceive the destruction of Israel as a catastrophe in which evil Arabs would throw the Jews into the sea. This is not a likely outcome. Before Zionism, Jews, Muslims and Christians coexisted relatively peacefully in Palestine for centuries. While Christianity may be a peaceful religion, throughout much of history Jews were better off living with Muslims than they were living with Christians. If Muslims' goal in life was to kill Jews, they would have exterminated the Palestinian Jews in 1914, when there were 600,000 Palestinian Muslims and only 60,000 Jews. In fact, according to Morris, in the 27 years ending in 1908 there were but 13 Jews killed by Arabs in Palestine, of which all but 4 were in the course of robberies or other crimes.(Morris 2001, p. 59) The evidence that Arabs and Jews can live together peacefully is all around us. Israel even has Palestinian Arabs in the government. There is nothing about Palestinian DNA that makes them hate Jews.

Yet some people look at the sample they have seen of Muslim behavior and think that Muslim inclinations toward Jews are reminiscent of Nazi Germany. Some call Iranian leader Ahmadinejad our modern-day Hitler. Throwing the word "Hitler" around shouldn't be done lightly. Ahmadinejad hasn't built any gas chambers. There's a significant Jewish community to this day in Iran. I don't know how free Iranian Jews feel they are to practice their Judaism[8], but there is no evidence to call Ahmadinejad a Hitler. On the contrary, perhaps he is right on the mark when he says that what the Germans did to the Jews does not justify what European Jews did to Palestinian people. "If you have burned the Jews, why don't you give a piece of Europe, the United States, Canada, or Alaska to Israel," Ahmadinejad said. "Our question is, if you have committed this huge crime, why should the innocent nation of Palestine pay for this crime" (CNN, 2005)?

We all hope the terrorism, the killing committed by both sides, comes to an end. We all want a just and peaceful solution. Some promote the idea of a separate Palestinian state as a means to that end, but if that solution doesn't allow Palestinian refugees the right to return to their homes, it won't solve the root cause of the conflict, nor would it be likely to end to the violence.

In his book, *One Country: A Bold Proposal to End the Israeli-Palestinian Impasse*, Palestinian American Ali Abunimah summarizes the problem (2006). He recounted the comments of the mother of a peace-activist friend. The mother was herself a refugee who had fled Germany in 1935 and whose comment presented the prevailing Zionist opinion.

"The State of Israel makes sure that next time we will not die unprotected, but with a rifle in our hand; for this reason, Jews cannot afford the luxury of understanding the Palestinian point of view." Such views, my friend

---

8. There are signs that the Iranian Jewish community is free to practice Judaism even while Iran makes anti-Zionist statements,(Demick, 2008)

was suggesting, are so deeply entrenched that there is simply no point challenging them. But one could argue that the most dangerous place in the world to be a Jew is in Israel-Palestine, and that this is the direct result of the conflict that arose from establishing a state that benefits and privileges Jews in a country already populated by a non-Jewish majority.

There are strong moral reasons not to accept the proposal that "Jews cannot afford the luxury of understanding the Palestinian point of view." The take-home lesson of the Holocaust is summarized on the final floor of the United States Holocaust Memorial Museum in Washington.

> First they came for the socialists, and I did not speak out—
> Because I was not a socialist.
> Then they came for the trade unionists, and I did not speak out—
> Because I was not a trade unionist.
> Then they came for the Jews, and I did not speak out—
> Because I was not a Jew.
> Then they came for me—and there was no one left to speak for me.
>
> —Attributed to Martin Niemöller (1892-1984),
> anti-Nazi German pastor

The lesson of the Holocaust was not every man was for himself; the lesson was our shared responsibility to human rights and dignity.

Abunimah speaks to the real goal of a one-state solution (2006). "The point," he says, "is not to deny Jews a safe haven in

Palestine-Israel, but to make the necessary changes that at last allow it to become one for the first time since Israel was founded." He laid out eight principles for a one-state solution, principles that would appeal to a Palestinian American or to a Jewish American or to a Christian American.

1. The power of the government shall be exercised with rigorous impartiality on behalf of all the people in the diversity of their identities and traditions and shall be founded on the principles of full respect for and quality of civil, political, social and cultural rights, and of freedom from discrimination for all citizens, women and men, and of parity of esteem and of just and equal treatment for the identity, ethos, and aspirations of all communities.

2. The constitution recognizes that the state is formed by the free and consenting union of two principal national communities, Israeli Jews and Palestinians, which each have multiple subcultures, shared histories, and sometimes irreconcilable narratives binding them to the country. Citizens of the state can call it a Jewish state or a Palestinian state if they wish to identify it as such. It will be both equally, simultaneously, and without contradiction. It is possible to be a full citizen of the state without belonging to either of these communities.

3. The state, recognizing the distinctive identities of the national communities who live in it, supports their linguistic and cultural traditions and production, all of which are part of the cultural wealth of the country. The state has mechanisms for national communities to exercise autonomy in decision-making related to language, educations, culture, and other matters, but which do not foster interethnic competition, discrimination, or separatism.

4. The state guarantees the freedom of religion and worship of every citizen and does not interfere in the affairs of religious communities. The state is neutral among religious groups and any state funding for religious schools or other institutions is distributed in a nondiscriminatory, transparent, and equitable manner.

5. While it is recognized that victims have a right to remember their history and to contribute to a changed society, the state enables all its citizens to participate in developing shared public spaces and symbols, as well as celebrations of common citizenship and identity that can be inclusive of people from every community.

6. The state recognizes that Israeli Jews have a special relation with Jewish communities outside the country, and that Palestinians and Israeli Jews of Arab origin are connected to the broader Arab world and to Arab diasporic communities, and that all are free to maintain and develop these vital relationships.

7. The state, recognizing that Israel-Palestine is a focus for adherents of the three monotheistic faiths all over the world, accepts that it has a special responsibility to ensure protection and access to all holy places.

8. The state actively fosters economic opportunity, social justice, and a dignified life for all its citizens, and establishes fair and efficient mechanism to compensate victims of the conflict and redress inequalities caused by unjust practices in the past.

Above all, Abunimah says that the Jews of Israel must be presented a vision that they would be protected in a single-state solution to the conflict. To do this, he says, the current state should be fought not by killing Israeli civilians but by resisting the morally bankrupt policies of the current government. The violence Israelis face only reinforces and perpetuates their fear of another Holocaust.

Abunimah sees the end of apartheid in South Africa as a successful model for ending conflict between Israelis and Palestinians. South Africa had Mandela offering white South Africans a vision of a peaceful future. Much as was the case in South Africa, ending Israeli fear will be difficult; ending Palestinian animosity would be much easier. Their violence and hatred would end if the Palestinian refugees were repatriated and treated as equals. Just ask Muslims, not Cal Thomas, how repatriating the Palestinians would change Palestinians' and other Muslims' views of Israel.

"Axis of Evil" or "the Great Satan"

Former President Bush called Iran part of an "axis of evil." Some Americans accept that and think Iran is the source of violence in the Middle East. John McCain, while campaigning before a group of American veterans, jokingly threatened to bomb Iran, singing, "that old Beach Boys song, Bomb Iran. Bomb, bomb, bomb, bomb," to the tune of the Beach Boys' song "Barbara Ann" (McCullagh 2008). On the other side, some Iranians have called the United States the Great Satan. People in each of these countries see themselves as in the right and see the other as downright evil. Surely someone has a misperception.

Why does it seem that so many Muslims hate us? We tell ourselves it is because they are jealous of our freedom. Does that make any sense at all? Is that what Iranians would say if we asked them? Not likely. Perhaps former Vice President Dick Cheney may not be the best person to ask if we want to understand how Iranians view Americans and why they see us the way they do. Iranians themselves might provide more reliable information on how Iranians actually think. One good source may be Shirin Ebadi.

Ms. Ebadi was the winner of the 2003 Nobel Peace prize. She won for courageous efforts in support of democracy and human rights, especially for the rights of women and children. Her book, *Iran Awakening: A Memoir of Revolution and Hope*, published in 2006, is a memoir describing her years before and after the Iranian Revolution (Ebadi 2006). The book is largely critical of Iran's fundamentalist Islamic government. Ebadi is a lawyer and was the first woman in the history of Iranian justice to have served as a judge. After the revolution, the Islamic Iranian government excluded women from being judges, making her a clerk in the court in which she formerly had been a judge. After regaining her license to practice law, she represented several journalists accused or sentenced in relation to freedom of expression.

Ms. Ebadi is not an apologist for the Iranian government. The Iranian government was at best lukewarm about her receiving the Nobel Prize and in part hostile. As an Iranian who is critical of Iran's Islamic government, Ms. Ebadi's harsh view of the United States ought to carry some weight.

According to Ebadi, Iranians' perceptions of their relationship with the United States have been shaped by U.S. intervention in Iran. In 1953, the United States was involved in the overthrow of the democratically elected prime minister of Iran, Mohammad Mosaddeq. Subsequently, the United States supported a dictator, the shah, over the Iranian people. When the Iranians threw out the dictator, relations with the United States soured. More recently, the United States supported Saddam Hussein in his war with Iran. The United States supported Hussein even while he was using nerve gas and later mustard gas on the Iranians. Hundreds of thousands of young Iranian men were killed in that war, changing the face of Iran for a generation. In her memoir, Ebadi describes in detail the horror of the mustard gas attacks and the impact of the huge numbers of casualties among the Iranians.

Now the United States has troops stationed in the country on Iran's eastern border, Iraq, and in the country on Iran's western border, Afghanistan. U.S. naval warships patrol the Persian Gulf off the southern coast of Iran. The U.S. government claims it is against Iran's nuclear program and proliferation of nuclear weapons in the Middle East, though the United States says nothing about the nuclear capabilities of Israel, a state Iranians perceive as created by largely European Zionists who displaced hundreds of thousands of Palestinian men, women, and children. The Iranians see the United States backing Israel even as Israel continues to kill more Palestinians and invades neighboring countries. Iranians heard the former President Bush threaten more economic sanctions against Iran and heard him talk of the potential for military strikes.

Is Iran part of an axis of evil? Within the minds of Iranian people, I doubt they would see it that way. Given the context in which they perceive the United States, is it unreasonable for them to believe that the United States government is the leader of an axis of evil? Given Carnegie's golden rule, one could see how they might perceive such a thing. With the context of past U.S.-Iranian relations in the minds of Iranian people, how should we expect Iranians to perceive us? As a beacon of freedom and democracy? Perhaps more likely they would see us as a colonial power trying to assert itself.

We see ourselves as a G-d-fearing, honest, hardworking, fair, and charitable people. We must think Iranians are stupid and evil when they call us the Great Satan. Yet former President Bush called Iran part of the "axis of evil" even though Iran never overthrew our leader, never installed a dictator over us, and never invaded our country. Iranians didn't support anyone using poison gases against us. Whatever the Iranians have done to us have paled in comparison to what we have done to them. If we can perceive Iran as evil on the basis of their actions, surely we ought to be able to see how Iranians might perceive us or our government as evil for our actions.

It isn't hard to understand their perspective if we try. The United States claims that Iran is interfering in Iraq. From their perspective, the United States is meddling in the Middle East. Iranian President Ahmadinejad responded to U.S. allegations that Iran was interfering by saying, "Is it not funny that those with 160,000 forces in Iraq accuse us of interference" (BBC News 2008)?

Iranian perspectives can also be seen in their response to President Obama's warm greetings to Iran sent at the time of the Persian New Year.(Wilayto 2009) In his message Obama said, "The United States wants the Islamic Republic of Iran to take its rightful place in the community of nations. You have that right—but it comes with real responsibilities, and that place cannot be reached through terror or arms, but rather through peaceful actions that demonstrate the true greatness of the Iranian people and civilization." We can expect Iranians to think that the greatness of the United States cannot be reached through terror or arms, too. Ayatollah Ali Khamenei, Iran's top religious leader and military commander-in-chief, responded to Obama saying that changes in U.S. actions are needed. Khamenei's complaints against the United States include 30 years of sanctions, seizure of Iranian assets, supporting Saddam Hussein's eight-year war with Iran, giving unconditional support for Israel, the killing of 300 civilians in the 1988 downing of an Iranian airplane by the USS Vincennes, and alleged U.S. support for anti-Iranian terrorist attacks along the Iran-Pakistan border. Iran has grievances with the United States, and they aren't about American freedom.

Iran is not a monolith. There appear to be conflicts between the people and the leadership there (almost undoubtedly they perceive the same thing about us, liking us as a people, but hating our government). Many Iranians find their government to be oppressive and would like to see greater tolerance of individual freedom. Some Iranians may believe their leadership is evil. But one should consider the possibility that those leaders—people who grew up seeing the United States support a dictator over them and who saw the United States supporting Saddam Hussein using poison gas on them—might have honest concerns that the United States is a threat to their country and that they must be prepared to meet that threat. Based on the things they've observed in their lives, perhaps their paranoia that we are against Islam is far more understandable (but still just paranoia) than our paranoia that they are against Christianity.

Iran has a lot going for it. The Iranian people aren't altogether different from us. Having met several Iranian dermatologists, one finds they are interested, peace loving, caring people, just like we are. The ones I've spoken with have been welcoming and seeking cordial relationships. One of them wrote to say,

> I believe that even true Muslims can live happily and in peace with their friends from other religions. My best friends in the University were three Jews and we're still good friends. Also, I have many American Jewish friends who all are nice guys.

In describing the government of Iran, he went on to declare,

> I don't want to say that we are smart or elegant people, but we had a revolution for our Constitution about one century ago and we had a National Assembly at that time when no other country in the region had one. Then, we had a desperate period after Mossadegh [the democratically elected leader overthrown by the United States], and finally we thought that the solution is mixing religion with politics. I accept that we had an obvious deterioration over a century.

Those who think that Iranians are inherently unfriendly or evil need to meet more Iranians.

One can and should wonder whether a small sample of Iranian dermatologists is representative of Iranian people in general. Jared Cohen, in his book, *Children of Jihad: A Young American's Travels among the Youth of the Middle East*, offers a much more intimate and detailed assessment of Iranian people (2007). In a truly remarkable journey, Cohen, an American Jew, travelled to Iran, Iraq, Syria, and Lebanon, meeting young people and delving into their experiences. Despite being open about being an American, he was welcomed and treated as a friend. In Iran, he found the system of government to be stifling, and he found young people chafing under its rules. Yet the young people he interacted with were no different from American young people—seeking new experiences, listening to music, interacting with each other, and pushing the limits that their society imposed. Many of the people he encountered expressed pro-American feelings while at the same time expressing the kind of pride in their own country that we have in ours.

Iranian expatriates may be in a good position to see both sides of the U.S.-Iran conflict. Robert Rezaei left his home in Iran in the 1970s and settled in San Antonio, Texas, (2007). He's lived in the Unites States for over thirty years and visits family and friends in Iran every three years. His parents still live in Shiraz, a city that is 2,500 years old, the former capital of the Persian Empire.

Robert has seen firsthand the terrible misconceptions people in the United States and in Iran have of each other. He finds that Americans' understanding of Iranians is very poor. Some Americans have asked him to denounce Iran. But Robert says Iranians are friendly, peace-loving people. Americans may see angry-looking Iranian protests with people shouting and carrying signs saying the Unites States is the Great Satan on the evening news. Robert says that while there is anger in Iran against the U.S. government, such protests aren't representative of the views most Iranians have of Americans. The views of most Iranians, spoken quietly, don't make the news.

Robert has also found that some Iranians have warped impressions of Americans. When visiting Iran, he sometimes has to dispel the notion that Americans have horns and tails. He understands why some Iranians might think this way. Iranians rarely get to see regular Americans, but when U.S. soldiers tortured Iraqis at Abu Graib, Robert says our mistreatment of Muslims was all-day, everyday, headline news in Iran. Robert works as a taxi driver. San Antonio is home to several large military bases, and Robert gets to drive American servicemen on a regular basis. He knows they are "just kids, trying to earn a living, trying to protect their country. They don't want to kill or torture anyone." Newspapers in Iran don't cover that side of things any more than U.S. news services cover all the friendly Iranians who respect Americans and who just want to see peace.

Robert says that when Americans visit Iran, they are treated as welcomed guests by Iranian people. That's what Norman Neureiter found on his visit to Iran (AAAS, 2007). Neureiter, director of the American Association for the Advancement of Science Center for Science, Technology, and Security Policy, attended an Iranian university reception for an American scientist. The scientist was treated as a celebrity. "It was phenomenally favorable, from the first day," he said. "It's amazing how popular Americans are in Iran. Intuitively, you would think it would be just the opposite." U.S. news media stories about Iran give us a very inaccurate impression of Iran and how friendly Iranians would be toward us.

Iranians may not like American policies, but they don't hate Americans and certainly aren't resentful of our freedom. Iranians take great pride in their culture. In particular, they take great pride in having given the world the first charter of human rights, and in having done so 1,500 years before the Europeans made a similar statement. The idea that they hate us for our freedom is ridiculous. Maybe our relationship with Iran would benefit from our leaders publicly admitting the extent of our past intrusions into Iranian affairs. Perhaps taking an attack on Iran off the table would be far more constructive than further threats. Ending the conflict with Iran ought to be very easy, considering how easy it would be to correct the misperceptions on which it is based.

Do similar principles tell us what we should be doing in Iraq? We've created a horrible mess there. Knowing how we would react to foreign power invading our country, perhaps there's no better solution than for us to get out and get out now. Adding in an apology wouldn't hurt. Perhaps I'm hopelessly naïve. But I fear that those who think things will get better the longer our army is there may be more naïve than I am.

Alternate Visions on how to End the Terrorism We Face

Compartments have powerful effects on our perceptions of the world. Acting on misguided perceptions can lead us horribly astray. Cal Thomas and Paul Craig Roberts showed us that there are at least two potential understandings of our relationship with the Muslim world. One holds that the Muslim world is evil and that the United States is the great beacon of freedom to the world. The other is that the Muslim world is no more evil than we are, and that many U.S. actions have been self-serving or at the very least misguided, particularly as perceived by people in the Muslim world. These two worldviews lead to very different views on how to end terrorism.

Much of our understanding of the Middle East and of our Middle East policies have been based on the assumptions that the United States has been blameless and justified in its actions and that the founding of Israel was done in a vacuum rather than at the expense of hundreds of thousands of Palestinian Arab inhabitants. While these assumptions were not made maliciously, they may have been about as accurate as dermatologists' understanding of patients' use of their medications. If U.S. actions were taken out of self-serving oil interests, if our support of Zionist Jews at the expense of Palestinian Arabs was misplaced, then much of the dogma about our relationship with the Middle East collapses like a house of cards, and an entirely different understanding emerges.

Based on the former assumptions, we have considered Iran to be an evil terrorist state and subjected them to sanctions. We consider bombing them too and perhaps even invading. If these policies are based on false assumptions, there may be far better ways to engage Iran. Perhaps we could admit publicly that the United States had the democratically elected prime minister of Iran overthrown in the 1950s and that we supported a dictator, the shah, there. We could apologize to Iranians for what role we had in the organization and support of the shah's secret police, the SAVAK. We could also apologize to Iran for supporting Saddam Hussein in his war against Iran and for turning a blind eye while Hussein used chemical weapons against the Iranian people. We could take force off the table as an option against Iran. Our past policies make a lot of sense under the ridiculous assumption that Iran is inherently evil. A new approach makes sense if Iranians are people who feel and act the way we do. Some would argue that it is naïve to think their culture is similar to ours. The best way to find out might be to visit Iran and get to know Iranians better. Depending on Christian or Jewish Americans for an understanding of Iranian Muslims is likely to be misleading.

The United States is deeply involved with many other primarily Muslim countries. In many of these countries, we support dictatorial regimes that act in accordance with our ends. Continuing to support dictators over people might seem to violate our own principles, but perhaps it makes sense if such dictators are needed to fight evil terrorism or if the people living in those countries are so different from us that they wouldn't know what to do with democracy if they had it. On the other hand, if what we perceive as evil terrorism represents people trying to fight the injustices that they perceive we have committed, maybe we are compounding the problem by supporting dictators over them. The people of these countries may be chafing under these oppressive dictatorships much as we would. Our support of their dictators probably doesn't help our reputation in their eyes. The actions we take that result from our misunderstanding of Muslims (misunderstanding that borders on paranoia) actually create the hate and violence we fear.

Our current dogma tells us to fight terrorism with violence and that appeasement of evil terrorists will only encourage the violence they commit. The dogma tells us to provide Israel military aid and diplomatic cover in the conflict with Palestinians, thinking that Israel is the only democracy in the Middle East. The dogma tells us it is appropriate to take any means necessary to stop any Middle East country other than Israel from developing atomic weapons. However, if we believe that it was wrong for 700,000 Arab people to be made refugees in order to create a state controlled by and for Jews, these policies would make little sense. To Muslim eyes, a country founded and run by and for Jews is no true democracy. The appeasement shoe would be on the other foot as Muslims would believe that any attempt at appeasing Israel would encourage her to take yet more land from Palestinian inhabitants. With a more balanced understanding of the cause of the Israel Palestinian conflict, we would see that the violence we support is counterproductive. Instead, we might start with an apology for supplying many of the weapons that have been used to kill Palestinian and Lebanese civilians. We could support the repatriation of Palestinian refugees into Israel, offering to help build homes instead of sending more F-16s or cluster bombs to Israel. We could establish relations with the democratically elected Palestinian leadership, even if they have committed acts of violence, recognizing that we don't have a problem with having

---

close relations with Israelis who committed acts of violence against Muslims. We could consider how it might appear hypocritical when we say we want to promote democracy while we turn our backs on democratically elected leaderships like that of Hamas. We might even announce a balanced policy on nuclear weapons in the Middle East that treats Iran and/or other Muslim countries and Israel equally in whatever moves are made to prevent nuclear proliferation.

If it is true that Jews created Israel in some completely blameless way, or if G-d selected the Jewish people to take Israel as some miracle, then perhaps continued unwavering support of Israel is sensible. If, however, the creation of the Jewish state was done at the expense of Palestinian Arabs, by the immoral destruction of entire Palestinian villages, then perhaps a change in our policies would be more in keeping with both our principles and our best interests.

Our previous assumptions tell us we should continue to fight terrorists with violence, killing terrorists until they are all dead, along with unavoidable, "accidental" collateral civilian deaths too. We have accepted that violence is the only thing these terrorists understand. However, if we change our understanding of how Israel was started, then all our concepts about which side has been committing the terrorism versus which side has been retaliating are turned upside down. If the violence we reap comes from the violence we sow, perhaps ending violence may be more productive than increasing it. We could suggest a complete and total amnesty for Palestinians considered guilty of terrorism, recognizing that the killing they have done is no better or worse than the killing the Israelis have done. If we feel the need to punish those who have blood on their hands, we would punish those who killed with crude bombs and those who killed using F-16s alike.

The idea that we must maintain or enlarge our armed presence in the Middle East is based on thinking that without our presence, evil and violence will continue to spread. Under a new set of assumptions, it might seem more appropriate to withdraw U.S. forces from the Middle East, thinking that we don't belong there any more than Iranian or Saudi armed forces belong in Canada or Mexico.

Whatever assumptions we make about our relationship with the Middle East, some things seem clear. We should wean ourselves from our oil/energy dependence either because we think it leaves us at the mercy of oil rich, evil Muslim countries or because if it weren't for our addiction to oil, we wouldn't be violating our own principles of freedom and democracy by supporting oppressive regimes in Muslim countries.

Our assumptions, our context, dramatically impact how we view the objective realities in the Middle East. Different assumptions lead to diametrically opposed directions for how we should interact with other people. One doesn't have to be evil or stupid or ignorant to favor one of these approaches over the other. Which view of the world one holds depends on one's experiences and how these experiences shape the perceptions we have of our observations. Unfortunately, our observations of the world can, at times, be very misleading.

President Barack Obama recognizes the misconceptions held by people on both sides of this conflict. Obama lived in Indonesia, the largest Muslim country. On January 27, 2009, in his first major interview after becoming president, he spoke to a reporter for the Al Arabiya network. In the interview, Obama said (Obama 2009):

> ... my job is to communicate to the American people
> that the Muslim world is filled with extraordinary
> people who simply want to live their lives and see their

179

children live better lives. My job to the Muslim world is to communicate that the Americans are not your enemy. We sometimes make mistakes. We have not been perfect. But if you look at the track record, as you say, America was not born as a colonial power, and that the same respect and partnership that America had with the Muslim world as recently as 20 or 30 years ago, there's no reason why we can't restore that. And that I think is going to be an important task.

. . . ultimately, people are going to judge me not by my words but by my actions and my administration's actions. And I think that what you will see over the next several years is that I'm not going to agree with everything that some Muslim leader may say, or what's on a television station in the Arab world—but I think that what you'll see is somebody who is listening, who is respectful, and who is trying to promote the interests not just of the United States, but also ordinary people who right now are suffering from poverty and a lack of opportunity. I want to make sure that I'm speaking to them, as well.

In working to reduce misconceptions between people, Obama may do more to reduce terrorism than any amount of torture ever could.

This book began with a description of a 1948 medical miracle, the development of cortisone. The discoverers were awarded the 1950 Nobel Prize in Medicine. The 1950 Nobel Peace Prize was awarded to African American Ralph Bunche for his work in negotiating the 1948 armistice agreements between Israel and Arab states.

—

Bunche was born in Detroit, Michigan, and was raised in Los Angeles (Nobel Lectures 1972). He attended the University of California at Los Angeles on an athletic scholarship and graduated summa cum laude, valedictorian of his class. He did graduate work at Harvard, travelling to Africa to study French rule in Togoland and Dahomey. Bunche served as chair of the Department of Political Science at Howard University from 1928 until 1950 and was active in the civil rights movement. He helped lead a civil rights march organized by Martin Luther King, Jr., in Montgomery, Alabama, and supported the National Association for the Advancement of Colored People (NAACP).

Bunche held several positions in the U.S. State Department with a focus on issues related to colonial affairs. From 1947 to 1949, Bunche worked on the conflict in Palestine for the United Nations (UN). He served as assistant to the UN Special Committee on Palestine, then as principal secretary of the UN Palestine Commission. Bunche became the chief aide to the UN mediator, the Swedish Count Folke Bernadotte. While working to achieve a peaceful settlement, Count Bernadotte was assassinated.[9] Bunche was named acting UN mediator on Palestine. After months of negotiation, Bunche secured armistice agreements between Israel and Arab States and secured for himself the Nobel Peace Prize.

Bunche said, "May there be, in our time, at long last, a world at peace in which we, the people, may for once begin to make full use of the great good that is in us." Sometimes it is difficult to see that great good. Because of compartments, we tend not to see each other's humanity. When we do observe people in other compartments, we often notice only the violent people, even when

---

[9]   Count Bernadotte was assassinated by members of LEHI, a Jewish terrorist organization led in part by future Israeli Prime Minister Yitzhak Shamir. (Wikipedia, Count Folke Bernadotte, 2008)

—

they are few in number. When we consider conflicts with others, we may observe objective realities, but we view them subjectively from our own context.

Bunche could see past those things, realizing people's shared essential goodness. "I . . . believe in the essential goodness of my fellow man, which leads me to believe that no problem of human relations is ever insoluble," Bunche said. We should remember that, even when our teachers and our observations tell us otherwise.

Epilogue

The themes of this book were presented in the form of the Livingood Lecture at the plenary session of the 2006 American Academy of Dermatology meeting. Thousands of dermatologists were in attendance. Two other lecturers presented as well. The academy collected feedback from the attendees. The three lectures were all well received. The Livingood Lecture received the highest score of all. Eighty-seven percent of the survey respondents considered the lecture outstanding. Several people offered written comment on the lecture. One said the talk was thought provoking and worthwhile, another that it was timely and appropriate, and yet another that the talk was superb. One even said the talk was tremendous and that "I have never had my mind stretched like that in such a short period of time." It was encouraging that after the lecture several people spoke to me saying how important it was to say these things. One dermatologist said that he and another dermatologist noted that all the political issues in dermatology that were talked about at the meeting were issues that depended on one's context and perception.

The feedback wasn't uniformly positive, though. The Livingood Lecture was the only one of the three plenary lectures to receive a score of zero on any of the surveys, which it did from three survey respondents. One respondent commented that the talk was terrible and inappropriate, another that it was a disgrace and an embarrassment. A few people approached me weeks later to say that the lecture was a travesty and an insult to Dr. Livingood's name.

One thing was clear, all these dermatologists, the ones who loved the lecture and the ones who hated it, attended the same lecture. Objectively, they all saw and heard the same thing. Yet their perceptions of the lecture were diametrically opposite. That was one of the central themes of the lecture: people can look at one objective reality and, based on the context they bring to it, perceive totally different things.

Giving the Clarence Livingood Lecture is a great honor. Traditionally, the lectures have been subsequently published in the *Journal of the American Academy of Dermatology*. The editor of the journal refused to consider a manuscript version of this Livingood Lecture for publication unless the political content was removed. In actuality, the whole lecture was, and this whole book is, political content. I asked the editor to reconsider, saying that restriction of the content of the article was an infringement of academic freedom. An independent reviewer of the article said he thought the political content in the article "was out there," but that academic freedom would not tolerate taking it out. The editor responded that there was no abridgement of academic freedom, that the author could freely submit the article to another journal. Two observers looked at the same manuscript and had diametrically opposed perceptions of whether it was an infringement of academic freedom to demand the political content to be removed prior to publication.

This book started by asking the question, is there an evil power underlying conflict in the world? And depending on how you look at it (and after reading this book you probably realize that "depending on how you look at it" isn't to be taken lightly), the answer is yes.

Satan, the evil power, is misunderstanding. Misunderstanding is built into the way our world is organized and structured. The compartments in which the world is organized are a feeding ground for misunderstandings that result in conflict. A world full of good people can still be a world troubled by conflict.

When we look at the conflicts in our own lives and in the world around us, we should ask ourselves if we really understand how others see things. Are there things that we are missing, things we aren't seeing that could explain the conflict? Are the things we are seeing representative, or are we just noticing a sample that doesn't accurately reflect the whole? Is it possible that the reason we saw something was *because* it wasn't representative of the norm? Finally, what we perceive as real, as true, as fact, depends on our context. We should ask, "What is the objective reality?" and we should ask whether others have reason to perceive it differently than we do. Where we stand depends on where we sit.

When we do these things, we may find that we have a lot in common with those we previously thought were our enemy. We may find that others are no more evil than we are. We may find ways to work more productively toward shared goals. We may even find a path to greater peace for ourselves and our children.

About the Author

Dr. Steven R. Feldman is a professor of dermatology, pathology, and public health sciences at the Wake Forest University School of Medicine in Winston-Salem, North Carolina. He was born in Washington, DC, and attended grade school at the Hebrew Academy of Washington, a school that his grandfather helped to found. His family was active in the orthodox Beth Shalom Synagogue where Feldman attended services and had his bar mitzvah.

Feldman received his bachelor's degree with a focus in chemistry at the University of Chicago. He received his MD and PhD degrees from Duke University in Durham, North Carolina, in 1985, following which he completed his dermatology residency at the University of North Carolina at Chapel Hill and his dermatopathology residency at the Medical University of South Carolina, in Charleston. Since 1991, he has been on the faculty at the Wake Forest University School of Medicine.

Dr. Feldman directs the Center for Dermatology Research, a health services research center whose mission is to improve the care of patients with skin disease. Dr. Feldman's chief clinical interest is psoriasis. His passion is to help guide how patients with psoriasis are treated. He served two terms as a member of the Medical Board of the National Psoriasis Foundation, chaired that board's subcommittee on education, and served as the director of the foundation's chief residents' meeting on psoriasis treatment from 2000 to 2005. He also served as chair of the American Academy of Dermatology's Psoriasis Education Initiative Workgroup, developing regional courses on emerging psoriasis therapies. Dr. Feldman was director of the psoriasis symposium at the 2005 and 2006 American Academy of Dermatology (AAD) Annual Meetings and is a frequent speaker to lay groups, physicians, industry professionals, and managed care executives. He received a Presidential Citation from the American Academy of Dermatology in 2005 for his psoriasis education efforts and received one of the AAD's highest awards, the Clarence S. Livingood Lecturership, at the 2006 AAD meeting.

Dr. Feldman has made significant contributions to understanding dermatologic health care delivery. His research team has focused on demonstrating the quality of medical dermatology services provided by dermatologists; defining the role of dermatologists in performing dermatopathology; assessing cost effectiveness of dermatologic treatments; and, most importantly, understanding the effectiveness, safety, and cost-effectiveness of outpatient dermatologic surgery. His research group has also published seminal studies on the dermatology workforce, the quality of life impact of psoriasis, and the reinforcing effects of UV exposure in frequent tanners. The work on tanning was covered extensively by major news media; Diane Sawyer interviewed Dr. Feldman concerning the implications of his tanning research on *Good Morning America*. Dr. Feldman's research studies into patients' compliance with their topical treatments helped transform how dermatologists understand and manipulate patients' use of topical medications over the course of chronic disease. Dr. Feldman was awarded the Astellas Award (and its $30,000 prize) by the

—

American Academy of Dermatology in 2008 for scientific research that improved public health in the field of dermatology.

Dr. Feldman founded the Medical Quality Enhancement Corporation and its www.DrScore.com Web site. The site is designed to help patients give doctors feedback so that doctors can enhance the quality of care they offer.

Dr. Feldman's work has been published in over 350 articles in peer-reviewed journals, including top-flight dermatology and managed care journals. He has been a primary investigator or coinvestigator on numerous industry, foundation, or federally funded research grants. Dr. Feldman has given over 600 invited lectures to dermatology groups and organizations. Since 1993, he has been a member of the editorial board of the *Journal of the American Academy of Dermatology*. He also serves as an editor of the *Journal of Dermatological Treatment*, on the editorial board of the *Journal of Cutaneous Medicine and Surgery* (the official publication of the Canadian Dermatology Association), the *Southern Medical Journal,* and *Dermatology Online Journal*, and as chief medical editor of *Skin & Aging*.

References

AAAS. In a time of tension, scientists build hopeful U.S.-Iran links. Science 2007:318:1886.

Abunimah A. *One Country: A Bold Proposal to End the Israeli-Palestinian Impasse*. Metropolitan Books, New York, New York, 2006.

Afrikaner Christianity: The Dutch Reformed Churches in South Africa. http://www.bethel.edu/~letnie/AfricanChristianity/SAAfrikanerChurches.html, accessed January 21, 2008.

Ali SM, Brodell RT, Balkrishnan R, Feldman SR. Poor adherence to treatments: a fundamental principle of dermatology. Arch Dermatol 2007;143:912-5.

American Academy of Dermatology. The Darker Side of Tanning. *http://www.aad.org/public/publications/pamphlets/sun_darker.html*. Accessed March 4, 2008.

American Academy of Dermatology Association. Indoor Tanning Fact Sheet. *http://www.dermexchange.com/media/background/factsheets/fact_indoortanning.html*. Accessed March 4, 2008.

BBC News. Iran leader in landmark Iraq trip. *http://news.bbc. co.uk/2/hi/middle_east/7273431.stm*. Accessed March 8, 2008.

Bush GW. Address to a Joint Session of Congress and the American People. *http://www.whitehouse.gov/news/ releases/2001/09/20010920-8.html*. Accessed February 10, 2008.

Carlin CS, Callis KP, Krueger GG. Efficacy of acitretin and commercial tanning bed therapy for psoriasis. Arch Dermatol 2003;139:436-42.

Carnegie D. *How to Make Friends and Influence People*. Pocket Books, 1990.

Carroll CL, Feldman SR, Camacho FT, Manuel JC, Balkrishnan R. Adherence to topical therapy decreases during the course of an 8-week psoriasis clinical trial: commonly used methods of measuring adherence to topical therapy overestimate actual use. J Am Acad Dermatol. 2004;51:212-6.

Christian Science Monitor. 'Why do they hate us?' *http://www. csmonitor.com/2001/0927/p1s1-wogi.html*. Accessed February 10, 2008.

City of Winston-Salem. Lee Garrity, City Manager. *http://www. ci.winston-salem.nc.us/Home/CityGovernment/CityManager/ Articles/LeeGarrity*. Accessed February 10, 2008.

CNN 2004. Bin Laden: 'Your security is in your own hands', *http://www. cnn.com/2004/WORLD/meast/10/29/bin.laden.transcript/*. Accessed February 10, 2008.

CNN 2005, Iranian leader: Holocaust a 'myth.' *http://www.cnn. com/2005/WORLD/meast/12/14/iran.israel/*, Accessed February 17, 2008.

CNN 2006. Moussaoui Gets Life; Was It Worth It? *http://transcripts. cnn.com/TRANSCRIPTS/0605/04/lt.01.html.* Accessed February 10, 2008.

Cohen J. *Children of Jihad: A Young American's Travels among the Youth of the Middle East.* Gotham, New York, New York, 2007.

Coldiron BM, Healy C, Bene NI. Office Surgery Incidents: What Seven Years of Florida Data Show Us. Dermatol Surg 2007.

Cordoro KM, Feldman SR. TNF-alpha inhibitors in dermatology. Skin Therapy Lett 2007;12:4-6.

De Jong R. Mega-Dose Lidocaine Dangers Seen in 'Tumescent' Liposuction. Anesthesia Patient Safety Foundation Newsletter 1999;14.

Demick B. Life of Jews Living in Iran: Iran remains home to Jewish enclave. *http://www.sephardicstudies.org/iran.html.* Accessed February 10, 2008.

Ebadi S. *Iran Awakening: A Memoir of Revolution and Hope.* Random House, New York, New York, 2006.

Epley N, Kruger J. When what you type isn't what they read: The perseverance of stereotypes and expectancies over e-mail. J Exp Soc Psych 2005;41:414-22.

Feldman SR. Looking beyond the borders of our specialty: The 2006 Clarence S. Livingood MD Lecture. Dermatology Online Journal 2007; 13: 20.

Feldman SR, Liguori A, Kucenic M, Rapp SR, Fleischer AB Jr, Lang W, Kaur M. Ultraviolet exposure is a reinforcing stimulus in frequent indoor tanners. J Am Acad Dermatol. 2004 Jul;51(1):45-51.

Fleischer AB Jr, Clark AR, Rapp SR, Reboussin DM, Feldman SR. Commercial tanning bed treatment is an effective psoriasis treatment: results from an uncontrolled clinical trial. J Invest Dermatol 1997;109:170-4.

Gilchrist A. Seeing in black & white: Why it isn't so cut-and-dried. Scientific American Mind 2006; June/July:42-9.

Giunca M. Moravians issue apology for church's role in slavery, Winston-Salem Journal, April 26, 2006.

Hamaker A. Personal Communication. 2008.

Hill MJ. iPLEDGE: protecting patients or prohibiting access to care? Dermatol Nurs 2006;18:124.

Hillhouse J, Turrisi R, Shields AL. Patterns of indoor tanning use: implications for clinical interventions. Arch Dermatol. 2007 Dec;143(12):1530-5.

Hurley HJ Jr, Strauss JS. Clarence S. Livingood, MD (1911-1998). Arch Dermatol 2000;136:1150-1151.

Kaur M, Liguori A, Fleischer AB Jr, Feldman SR. Side effects of naltrexone observed in frequent tanners: could frequent tanners have ultraviolet-induced high opioid levels? J Am Acad Dermatol. 2005 May;52(5):916.

Kaur M, Liguori A, Lang W, Rapp SR, Fleischer AB Jr, Feldman SR. Induction of withdrawal-like symptoms in a small randomized, controlled trial of opioid blockade in frequent tanners. J Am Acad Dermatol. 2006 Apr;54(4):709-11.

Kendall EC. Hormones of the adrenal cortex. Bull N Y Acad Med. 1953;29:91-100.

Krejci-Manwaring J, Tusa MG, Carroll C, Camacho F, Kaur M, Carr D, Fleischer AB Jr, Balkrishnan R, Feldman SR. Stealth monitoring of adherence to topical medication: adherence is very poor in children with atopic dermatitis. J Am Acad Dermatol. 2007;56:211-6.

Kruger J, Epley N, Parker J, Ng Z-W. Egocentrism over e-mail: Can we communicate as well as we think? J Personality Soc Psych 2005; 89: 925-36.

Kweder SL. Drug regulation in controversy: Vioxx. *www.fda.gov/cder/drug/infopage/vioxx/Vioxx_Kweder_20041110.ppt. Accessed February 19*, 2008.

Mawn VB, Fleischer AB Jr. A survey of attitudes, beliefs, and behavior regarding tanning bed use, sunbathing, and sunscreen use. J Am Acad Dermatol. 1993 Dec;29(6):959-62.

—

McCullagh D. YouTube deletes video of McCain singing 'Bomb Iran.' *http://news.cnet.com/2100-1025_3-6178173.html*, accessed October 12, 2008.

Mearshimer J. Disturbing debate. University of Chicago Magazine. 2006; 98: *http://magazine.uchicago.edu/0608/issue/letters.shtml*. Accessed February 10, 2008.

Menter MA. Martin Alan Menter, MD: a conversation with the editor. Interview by William

Clifford Roberts. Proc (Bayl Univ Med Cent) 2003;16:174-92.

Middle East Web. Israel and Palestine: A Brief History. *http://www.mideastweb.org/briefhistory.htm*. Accessed February 10, 2008.

Middle East Web. Plan Dalet. *http://www.mideastweb.org/pland.htm*. Accessed February 10, 2008.

Moravian Church of North America. *http://www.moravian.org/*. Accessed February 10, 2008.

Morell RC. OBA Questions, Problems Just Now Recognized, Being Defined. Anesthesia Patient Safety Foundation Newsletter 2000; 15.

Morris B. *Righteous Victims: A history of the Zionist-Arab conflict 1881-2001.*Vintage Books, New York, New York, 2001.

Moss E. Implementing OBA Regulations a Complex, Difficult Process. Anesthesia Patient Safety Foundation Newsletter 2000; 15.

National Public Radio, Morning Edition. Analysis: New England Journal of Medicine raises questions about the safety of liposuction. May 13, 1999.

Nelms H. *Magic and Showmanship: A Handbook for Conjurers.* Mineola, New York: Dover Publications, Inc, 1969.

Nobel Lectures, Peace 1926-1950, Editor Frederick W. Haberman, Elsevier Publishing Company, Amsterdam, 1972.

Obama B. Obama's interview with Al Arabiya. *http://www.alarabiya. net/articles/2009/01/27/65096.html. Accessed March 31*, 2009.

Old Salem Museum and Gardens. *http://www.oldsalem.org/.* Accessed February 10, 2007.

Proactiv. *http://www.proactiv.com/.* Accessed February 10, 2007.

Rao RB, Ely SF, Hoffman RS. Deaths related to liposuction. N Engl J Med 1999;340:1471-5.

Rezaei R. Personal communication, 2008.

Resneck JS Jr, Lipton S, Pletcher MJ. Short wait times for patients seeking cosmetic botulinum toxin appointments with dermatologists. J Am Acad Dermatol. 2007 Dec;57(6):985-9.

Roberts PC. Bringing Death and Destruction to Muslims. *http://www. antiwar.com/roberts/?articleid=12224.* Accessed February 10, 2008.

Seely H. The Poetry of D.H. Rumsfeld. Slate. *http://www.slate.com/ id/2081042/.* Accessed February 10, 2008.

Shavit A. Survival of the Fitest. Interview with Benny Morris. *Ha'aretz*, August 1, 2004, *http://www.haaretz.com/hasen/pages/ShArt. jhtml?itemNo=380986&sw=Beni%20Morris*, accessed February 20, 2009.

Shlaim A. *The Iron Wall: Israel and the Arab World*. WW Norton & Company, New York, New York, 2001.

Stern RS. Dermatologists in the year 2000: Will supply exceed demand? Arch Dermatol 1986;122:675-678.

Suren-Pahlav S. Cyrus Charter of Human Rights. Iran Chamber Society. *http://www.iranchamber.com/history/cyrus/cyrus_charter. php*. Accessed February 10, 2008.

Teaching Company. Great World Religions. *www.teach12.com*. Accessed February 17, 2008.

Thomas C. Misplaced Faith. *http://www.calthomas.com/index. php?news=2156*. Accessed February 10, 2008.

U.S. Department of Justice, Federal Bureau of Investigation. Crime Statistics in the United States, 2005, Table 1. *http://www.fbi.gov/ ucr/05cius/data/table_01.html*. Accessed February 10, 2008.

Venkat AP, Coldiron B, Balkrishnan R, Camacho F, Hancox JG, Fleischer AB Jr, Feldman SR. Lower adverse event and mortality rates in physician offices compared with ambulatory surgery centers: a reappraisal of Florida adverse event data. Dermatol Surg 2004;30:1444-51.

Vila H Jr, Soto R, Cantor AB, Mackey D. Comparative outcomes analysis of procedures performed in physician offices and ambulatory surgery centers. Arch Surg 2003;138:991-5.

Warthan MM, Uchida T, Wagner RF Jr. UV light tanning as a type of substance-related disorder. Arch Dermatol. 2005 Aug;141(8):963-6.

Wikipedia, Cal Thomas, *http://en.wikipedia.org/wiki/Cal_Thomas*. Accessed February 10, 2008.

Wikipedia, Count Folke Bernadotte of Wisborg. *http://en.wikipedia.org/wiki/Folke_Bernadotte*. Accessed February 10, 2008.

Wikipedia, Gilad Shalit. *http://en.wikipedia.org/wiki/Gilad_Shalit*. Accessed February 10, 2008.

Wikipedia. Going Postal. *http://en.wikipedia.org/wiki/Going_postal*. Accessed February 10, 2008.

Wikipedia. 1929 Hebron Massacre. *http://en.wikipedia.org/wiki/1929_Hebron_massacre*. Accessed February 10, 2008.

Wikipedia, Paul Craig Roberts. *http://en.wikipedia.org/wiki/Paul_Craig_Roberts*. Accessed February 10, 2008.

Wilayto P. Did Iran reject Obama's overture? *http://www.defendersfje.org/id18.html. Accessed March 31*, 2009.

Wintzen M, Yaar M, Burbach JP, Gilchrest BA. Proopiomelanocortin gene product regulation in keratinocytes. J Invest Dermatol. 1996 Apr;106(4):673-8.

Zimmerman G. Personal communication, January, 2007.

Index